Update on

Textbook of
Community Medicine

Preventive and Social Medicine | Fifth Edition

with Recent Advances

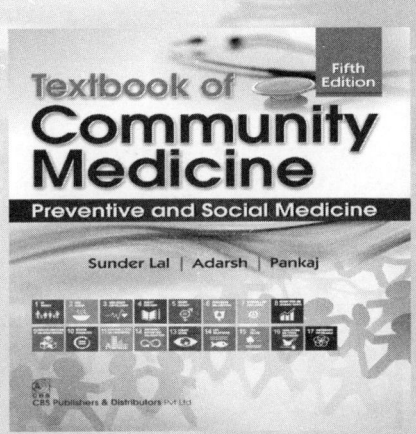

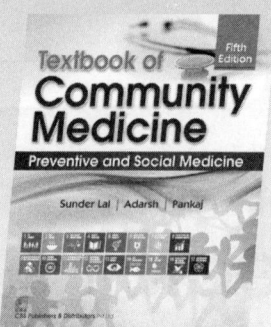

Update on

Textbook of
Community Medicine
| Preventive and Social Medicine | Fifth Edition

with Recent Advances

Dr (Brig) **Sunder Lal** MBBS, DPH, MD

Former
Professor and Head, Department of Social and Preventive Medicine
Pt BD Sharma Postgraduate Institute of Medical Sciences, Rohtak, Haryana
and AIMSR, Bathinda, Punjab
Professor, Department of Community Medicine, MM University, Mullana, Ambala
Deputy Director-General, TA (Medical)
Chairman, Board of Studies of Medicine and Allied Sciences, MDU, Rohtak
Member, National Commission on Population, GoI; Consultant, ICDS
Member, National Technical Advisory Group on Immunization and Child Health
Member, Technical Resource Group on Women, Children and ICDS
NSS Programme Officer
Honorary Professor, IMACGP, and
President of IAPSM

Adarsh MBBS

Former
Senior Medical Officer, HCMS (I)
Medical Officer-incharge, Postpartum Centre, PGIMS, Rohtak
Medical Officer-incharge, Urban Family Welfare Centre, Rohtak
Urban Health Centre attached with PGIMS, Rohtak, Haryana

Pankaj MDS

Ex-Professor, Department of Public Health Dentistry
Rajasthan Dental College, Jaipur, Rajasthan

CBS

CBS Publishers & Distributors Pvt Ltd

New Delhi • Bengaluru • Chennai • Kochi • Kolkata • Mumbai
Hyderabad • Jharkhand • Nagpur • Patna • Pune • Uttarakhand

Disclaimer

Science and technology are constantly changing fields. New research and experience broaden the scope of information and knowledge. The authors have tried their best in giving information available to them while preparing the material for this book. Although, all efforts have been made to ensure optimum accuracy of the material, yet it is quite possible some errors might have been left uncorrected. The publisher, printer and the authors will not be held responsible for any inadvertent errors, omissions or inaccuracies.

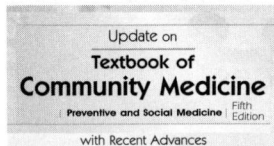

Update on

Textbook of

Community Medicine
Preventive and Social Medicine | Fifth Edition

with Recent Advances

ISBN: 978-93-87085-95-4

Copyright © Authors and Publisher

First Edition: 2018

All rights reserved. No part of this book may be reproduced or transmitted in any form or by any means, electronic or mechanical, including photocopying, recording, or any information storage and retrieval system without permission, in writing, from the authors and the publisher.

Published by Satish Kumar Jain and produced by Varun Jain for

CBS Publishers & Distributors Pvt Ltd

4819/XI Prahlad Street, 24 Ansari Road, Daryaganj, New Delhi 110 002, India.

Ph: 23289259, 23266861, 23266867   Website: www.cbspd.com

Fax: 011-23243014   e-mail: delhi@cbspd.com; cbspubs@airtelmail.in.

Corporate Office: 204 FIE, Industrial Area, Patparganj, Delhi 110 092

Ph: 4934 4934   Fax: 4934 4935   e-mail: publishing@cbspd.com; publicity@cbspd.com

Branches

- **Bengaluru:** Seema House 2975, 17th Cross, K.R. Road, Banasankari 2nd Stage, Bengaluru 560 070, Karnataka
  Ph: +91-80-26771678/79   Fax: +91-80-26771680   e-mail: bangalore@cbspd.com
- **Chennai:** 7, Subbaraya Street, Shenoy Nagar, Chennai 600 030, Tamil Nadu
  Ph: +91-44-26680620, 26681266   Fax: +91-44-42032115   e-mail: chennai@cbspd.com
- **Kochi:** Ashana House, No. 39/1904, AM Thomas Road, Valanjambalam, Ernakulam 682 016, Kochi, Kerala
  Ph: +91-484-4059061-65   Fax: +91-484-4059065   e-mail: kochi@cbspd.com
- **Kolkata:** 6/B, Ground Floor, Rameswar Shaw Road, Kolkata-700 014, West Bengal
  Ph: +91-33-22891126, 22891127, 22891128   e-mail: kolkata@cbspd.com
- **Mumbai:** 83-C, Dr E Moses Road, Worli, Mumbai-400018, Maharashtra
  Ph: +91-22-24902340/41   Fax: +91-22-24902342   e-mail: mumbai@cbspd.com

Representatives

- **Hyderabad** 0-9885175004 • **Jharkhand** 0-9811541605 • **Nagpur**   0-9021734563
- **Patna**   0-9334159340 • **Pune**   0-9623451994 • **Uttarakhand** 0-9716462459

Printed at Rashtriya Printers, Dilshad Garden, Delhi, India

Foreword

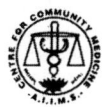

अखिल भारतीय आयुर्विज्ञान संस्थान
ALL INDIA INSTITUTE OF MEDICAL SCIENCES

डॉ चन्द्रकान्त एस पांडव
एम बी बी एस, एम डी (एम्स)
एम एम सी (मैक्मास्टर युनिवर्सिटी, कनाडा) एफ ए एम एस
आचार्य एवं विभागाध्यक्ष
सामुदायिक चिकित्सा केन्द्र
अंसारी नगर, नई दिल्ली 110029, भारत
फोन : 91-11-26588522, 26593553
फैक्स : 91-11-26588522

Dr. Chandrakant S. Pandav
MBBS, MD (AIIMS)
M.Sc. (McMaster Univ. Canada), FAMS
Professor and Head
Center for Community Medicine
Ansari Nagar, New Delhi-110029, India
Phone: 91-11-26588522, 26593553 Fax: 91-11-26588522
E-mail : cpandav@iqplusin.org.cpandav@indiatimes.com

It is a matter of great privilege for me to write the Foreword on update and recent advances of the fifth edition of *Textbook of Community Medicine* by Prof (Dr) Sunder Lal and coauthors (Dr Adarsh and Dr Pankaj). It is a unique book that not only imparts theoretical concepts but also lays emphasis on the applied and practical aspects of the preventive, promotive and curative health. This book fulfils the tenets of Miller's triangle in developing competence in community medicine in terms of *knows, knows how, shows how* and *does*. While being precise, the book has not compromised with the essential information.

Immense popularity of earlier editions, especially among students of community medicine, and the everchanging public health scenario in the country, have made it necessary to revise and update the earlier edition to suit the present-day requirements. Authors have incorporated all the recent developments in the field of community medicine and have been successful in presenting the information in lucid manner. Authors have also adhered to the current global trend in medical education of integration of clinical disciplines with preventive medicine with the focus of the integrated information on primary health care. This will provide proper perspective to the readers of the book.

I hope that this book will be of a great interest and use equally to students as well as professionals of community medicine and public health. I am quite confident that this book will be widely referred to and will be put into practice. I hope that like previous editions, this edition will also be a great success.

I congratulate the authors for bringing out the **update** on the fifth edition of *Textbook of Community Medicine*.

Chandrakant S Pandav

Preface

The update and recent advances in community medicine up to 2017 has been a necessity in view of evolution and fast track changes/approaches on the subject. Wide ranging advances have occured in the country as a result of sustainable development goals and thrust areas of NCDs. To club the learning resource material on recent developments at one place is essential to grasp the things quickly. Authors have made an effort to consolidate the material from different areas and programmes to enrich the text of 5th edition of community medicine. For more details the recent advances can be linked to whole text in respective chapters, specifically referred pages of respective chapters to get a comprehensive view on the subject special features.

Learning resource material incorporates Mandate of Medical Council of India, NFHS 4, NHP 2017, life saving commodities, national guidelines on STI/RTI 2014, National Health Accounts, NITI Aayog, health financing in India, integrated health management information system, April 2017, vision 2020 in FP, end TB strategies, 90; 90; 90 treatment goal in HIV, non-communicable diseases (population-based screening programme), ICMR, PHFI, and/HME 1990 to 2016 as a part of Global Disease Burden Study. Mental health survey 2015–16 and Mental Health Act 2017, linked confidential testing in HIV 2017, Malaria Elimination Plan 2017, newer vaccines, elimination of parent to child transmission of syphilis and HIV, BMI norms for Indian population, new estimates of blindness in India, trachoma elimination, food fortification, national immunization schedule, GATS 2016–17, neglected tropical diseases and mother's absolute affection (MAA) programme are significant areas. National Nutrition Mission 2017, National Strategic Plan and 'Mission Sampark' 2017 to 2024, vaccine against leprosy, dengue fever and changes in ESIS, kilkari programme and longitudinal ageing study in India have also been added as recent advances.

Sunder Lal
Adarsh
Pankaj

Acknowledgements

This update was made possible with the advice and contribution of many people. Help and guidance received from Dr Rajesh Kumar, Professor and Head, Department of Community Medicine, and Dean, PGIMER, Chandigarh; Dr Ajay Khera, DC, Child Health and Immunization; Dr D Bachani, DC, NCD; Dr Sunil D Khaparde, DDG, Central TB Division, Nirman Bhavan, New Delhi, Dr Anurag Chaudhary, Professor and Head, and Prof Sarit Sharma of DMC, Ludhiana (Punjab); Dr Manish Goyal, Associate Professor, LHMC; Dr Shanker Prinja, Associate Professor, PGIMER, Chandigarh; and Dr Kuldip Shingh, Civil Surgeon, Yamuna Nagar, Haryana, is sincerely acknowledged. The authors owe deep sense of gratitude to the World Health Organization (WHO), UNICEF, DGHS, Nirman Bhavan, and Ministry of Health and Family Welfare, ICMR, PHFI, and IHME whose published material has been used extensively to update and enrich the contents of text material for dissemination of scientific information to the students and teachers of community medicine.

Sunder Lal
Adarsh
Pankaj

Contents

Chapter numbers and titles given in this table of contents
correspond to the following book by the same authors:

Textbook of
Community Medicine
| Preventive Medicine |
Fifth Edition

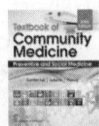

Abbreviations

ACD	Active case dectection
ACDR	Annual case detection rate
AEFI	Adverse event following immunization
AHS	Annual health survey
AIDS	Aquired immunodeficiency syndrome
Aliquot	Part of blood sample
ANC	Antenatal care
ANM	Auxilliary nurse midwife
API	Annual parasite incidence
ASHA	Accredited social health activisit
AYUSH	Ayurveda, Yoga Unani, Sidha and Homeopathy
CBNAAT	Cartridge based nucleic acid amplification test
CCD	Communicable diseases
COPD	Chronic obstructive pulmonary disease
CP	Continuation phase
CPHC	Comprehensive primary health care
CVDs	Cardio-vascular diseases
CXR	Chest X-ray
DALY	Disability adjusted life years
DBS	Dried blood spot
DEIC	District early intervention centre
DLHS	District level household survey
DM	Diabetes mellitus
DOTS	Directly observed treatment short course

DRTB	Drug resistant TB
DSTB	Drug sensitive TB
ESIS	Employee State Insurance Scheme
fIPV	Fractional inactivated polio vaccine
FP	Family planning
GATS	Global adult tobacco survey
GLV	Green leafy vegetables
Hb	Haemoglobin
HDL	High density lipids
HH	Household
HIb	Haemophilus influenzae type B
HIV	Human immunodeficiency virus
HMIS	Health management information system
HRG	High risk groups
HSS	HIV sentinel surveillance
IBBS	Integrated bio-behavioural surveillance
ICDS	Integrated Child Development Services Scheme
ICMR	Indian Council of Medical Research
IHD	Ischaemic heart disease
IHME	Institue for health metrics and evaluation
IMNCI	Integrated management of neo-natal and childhood illness
IMR	Infant mortality rate
IP	Intensive phase
IPHS	Indian public health standards
IUCD	Intrauterine contraceptive device
IUGR	Intrauterine growth retardation
IYCFP	Infant and young child feeding practices
JSY	Janani Suraksha Yojna
LPA	Line probe assay

MAA	Mother's absolute affection
MCH	Maternal and child health
MCI	Medical Council of India
MDA	Mass drug administration
MDR TB	Multi-drug resistant TB
MMR	Maternal mortality ratio
MOHFW	Ministry of health and family welfare
MR	Measles rubella
MTB	Mycobacterium tuberculosis
NCDs	Non communicable diseases
NCMH	National Commission on Macroeconomics and Health
NFHS-4	National family health survey 4
NHA	National Health Accounts
NHM	National Health Mission
NHP	National Health Policy
NIN	National Institute of Nutrition
NNM	National Nutrition Mission
NSS	National Sample Survey
NTDs	Neglected tropical diseases
OOPE	Out of pocket expenditure
PCD	Passive case detection
PCV	Pneumococcal conjugate vaccine
PHC	Primary health centre
PHFI	Public Health Foundation of India
PL HIV	Person living with HIV/AIDS
PMDT	Programmatic management of drug resistant TB
PNC	Postnatal care
PPIUCD	Post-partum IUCD
PPTCT	Prevention of parent to child transmission

PR	Prevalence rate
PTB	Pulmonary tuberculosis
RBSK	Rashtriya Bal Swasthya Karyakram
Rif	Rifampicin
RMNCH + A	Reproductive maternal newborn and child health + adslestent
RNTCP	Revised National TB Control Programme
SC	Subcentre
SDG	Sustainable development goals
SGA	Small for gestational age
STD	Sexually transmitted diseases
STI	Sexually tranmitted infection
TAS	Transmission Assessment Survey
U5 MR	Under five mortality rate
UHC	Urban health centre
Un HC	Universal health coverage
UN	United Nations
USHA	Urban social health activist
USI	Universal salt iodation
VLD	Very low density lipid
WHO	World Health Organization
XDRTB	Extensive drug resistant TB
ZN	Zeihl-Neelson

1

Orientation to Community Medicine, Social and Behavioural Sciences

MEDICAL COUNCIL OF INDIA REGULATIONS—AMENDED UP TO MARCH 2017

1. GENERAL CONSIDERATIONS AND TEACHING APPROACH

1. Graduate medical curriculum is oriented towards training students to undertake the responsibilities of a physician of first contact who is capable of looking after the preventive, promotive, curative and rehabilitative aspects of medicine.

2. With wide range of career opportunities available today, a graduate has a wide choice of career opportunities. The training, though broad based and flexible should aim to provide an education experience of the essentials required for health care in our country.

   The folllowing words have been added after sub-clause 2 after the words "care in our country" in terms of notification published on 15.12.2008.

   "Training should be able to meet internationally acceptable standards."

3. To undertake the responsibilities of service situations which is a changing condition and of various types, it is essential to provide adequate placement training tailored to the needs of such services as to enable the graduates to become effective instruments of implementation of those requirements. To avail of opportunities and be able to conduct professional requirements, the graduate shall endeavour to have acquired basic training in different aspects of medical care.

4. The importance of the **community aspects of health care** and of **rural health** care services is to be recognized. This aspect of education and training of graduates should be adequately

recognized in the prescribed curriculum. Its importance has been systematically upgraded over the past years and adequate exposure to such experiences should be available throughout all the three phases of education and training. This has to be further emphasized and intensified by providing exposure to field practice areas and training during the internship period. The aim of the period of rural training during internship is to enable the fresh graduates to function efficiently under such settings.

5. The educational experience should emphasize **health** and **community orientation** instead of only disease and hospital orientation or being concentrated on curative aspects. As such all the basic concepts of modern scientific medical education are to be adequately dealt with.

6. There must be enough experiences to be provided for self learning. The methods and techniques that would ensure this must become a part of teaching-learning process.

7. The medical graduate of modern scientific medicine shall endeavour to become capable of functioning independently in both urban or rural environment. He/she shall endeavour to give emphasis on fundamental aspects of the subjects taught and on common problems of health and disease avoiding unnecessary details of specialization.

8. The importance of **social factors** in relation to the problem of **health** and **diseases** should receive proper emphasis throughout the course and to achieve this purpose, the educational process should also be **community based** than **only hospital** based. The importance of population control and family welfare planning should be emphasized throughout the period of trainng with the importance of health and development duly emphasized.

9. Adequate emphasis is to be placed on cultivating logical and scientific habits of thought, clarity of expression and independence of judgement, ability to collect and analyse information and to correlate them.

10. The educational process should be placed in a historic background as an evolving process and not merely as an acquisition of a large number of disjointed facts without a proper perspective. The history of medicine with reference to the evolution of medical knowledge both in this country and the rest of the world should form a part of this process.

11. Lectures alone are generally not adequate as a **method of training** and are a poor means of transferring/acquiring

information and even less effective at **skill development** and in generating the appropriate attitudes. Every effort should be made to encourage the use of active methods related to demonstration and on first hand experience. Students will be encouraged to learn in small groups, through peer interactions so as to gain maximal experience through **contacts with** patients and the **communities** in which they live. While the curriculum objectives often refer to areas of knowledge or science, they are best taught in a setting of clinical relevance and hands on experience for students who assimilate and make this knowledge a part of their own working skills.

12. The graduate medical **education in** clinical subjects should be based primarily on out-patient teaching, emergency departments and **within the community** including peripheral health care institutions. The out-patient departments should be suitably planned to provide training to graduates in small groups.

13. Clinics should be organised in small groups of preferably not more than 10 students so that a teacher can give personal attention to each student with a view to improve his skill and competence in handling of the patients.

14. Proper records of the work should be maintained which will form the basis for the studnets' internal assessment and should be available to the inspectors at the time of inspection of the college by the Medical Council of India.

15. Maximal efforts have to be made to encourage **integrated teaching** between traditional subject areas using a **problem based learning approach** starting with clinical or community cases and exloring the relevance of various preclinical disciplines in both understanding and resolution of the problem. Every attempt be made to de-emphasize compartmentalisation of disciplines so as to achieve both horizontal and vertical integration in different phases.

16. Every attempt is to be made to encourage students to participate in group discussions and seminars to enable them to develop personality, character expression and other faculties which are necessary for a medical graduate to function either in solo practice or as a team leader when he begins his independent career. A discussion group should not have more than 20 students.

17. Faculty member should avail of modern educational technology while teaching the students and to attain this objective, Medical Education Units/Departments be established in all medical

colleges for faculty development and providing learning resource material to teachers.

18. To derive maximum advantage out of this revised curriculum, the vacation period to students in one calendar year should not exceed one month, during the 4½ years Bachelor of Medicine and Bachelor of Surgery (MBBS) Course.

19. In order to implement the revised curriculum in toto, State Govts and Institution Bodies must ensure that adequate financial and technical inputs are provided.

The following have been added after sub-clause 19 in terms of notification published on 15.12.2008 in the Gazette of India.

20. **History of medicine:** The students will be given an outline on 'History of Medicine'. This will be taught in an integrated manner by subject specialists and will be coordinated by the Medical Eduation Unit of the College.

21. All medical institutions should have curriculum committee which sould plan curricula and instructional method which will be regularly updated.

22. Integration of ICT in learning process will be implemented.

3. OBJECTIVE OF MEDICAL GRADUATE TRAINING PROGRAMME

I. **National Goals:** At the end of undergraduate program, the medical student should be able to:

a. Recognize 'health for all' as a national goal and health right of all citizens and by undergoing training for medical profession fulfill his/her social obligations towards realization of this goal.

b. Learn every aspect of **National policies** on **health** and devote himself/herself to its practical implementation.

c. Achieve competence in practice of holistic medicine, encompassing promotive, preventive, curative and rehabilitative aspects of common diseases.

d. Develop **scientific temper,** acquire educational experience for proficiency in profession and promote healthy living.

e. Become exemplary citizen by observation of **medical ethics** and fulfilling social and professional obligations, so as to respond to national aspirations.

II. **Institutional Goals**

I. In consonance with the national golas each medical institution should evolve institutional golas to define the kind of trained manpower (or professionals) they intend to produce. The undergraduate students coming out of a medical institute should:

a. Be competent in diagnosis and management of common health problems of the individual and the community, commensurate with his/her position as a member of the health team at the primary, secondary or tertiary levels, using his/her clinical skills based on history, physical examination and relevant investigations.

b. Be competent to practice preventive, promotive, curative and rehabilitative medicine in respect to the commonly encountered health problems.

c. Apprieciate rationale for different therapeutic modalities, be familiar with the administration of the "essential drugs" and their common side effects.

d. Be able to appreciate the **socio-psychological, cultural, economic** and **environmental factors affecting health** and develop **humane attitude** towards the patients in discharging one's professional responsibilities.

e. Possess the attitude for continued self learning and to seek further expertise or to pursue research in any chosen area of medicine.

The above sub-clause II(e) has been substituted in terms of notification published on 15.12.2008 in the Gazette of India and the same is as under:

e. Possess the attitude for continued self learning and to seek further expertise or to **pursue research** in any chosen area of medicine, **action research** and documentation skills.

f. *Be familiar with the basic factors which are essential for the implementation of the National Health Programmes including practical aspects of the following:*

i. Family Welfare and Material and Child Health (MCH)

ii. Sanitation and water supply

iii. Preventaion and control of communicable and non-communicable diseases.

iv. Immunization

v. Health education

The following have been added after sub-clause II(f)(v) in terms of notification published on 15.12.2008 in the Gazette of India.

vi. IPHS standard of health at various level of service delivery, medical waste disposal.

vii. Organisational institutional arrangements.

g. Aquire basic management skills in the area of human resource, material and resource management related to health care delivery.

The above sub-caluse 3(II)(g) has been substituted in terms of notification publised on 15.12.2008 in the Gazette of India and the same is as under:

g. Acquire **basic management skills** in the **area of human resources, materials** and **resource management related** to **health care delivery, General** and **hospital** management, principal inventory skills and counselling.

h. Be able to **identify community helath problems** and **learn to** work **to resolve** these by **designing,** instituting corrective steps and evaluating outcome of such measures.

i. Be able to work as a **leading** partner in **health care teams and** acquire proficiency in **communication skills.**
   - Be competent to work in a variety of health care settings.
   - Have personal characteristics and attitudes required for professional life such as personal integrity, sense of responsibility and dependability and ability to relate to or show concern for other individuals.

II. All efforts must be made to equip the medical graduate to acquire the skills as detailed in Appendix B.

4. INTRODUCTION TO HUMANITIES AND COMMUNITY MEDICINE

Including introduction to the **subjects of Demography, Health Economics, Medical Sociology, Hospital Management, Behavioural Sciences inclusive of Psychology.**

Objectives
a. Knowledge
The shudent shall be able to:

1. Explain the principles of sociology including **demographic population dynamics**.
2. Identify social **factors related to health disease** and **disability** in the context of urban and rural societies.
3. Appreciate the impact of **urbanization** on health and diseases.
4. Observe and interpret the dynamics of community behavior.
5. Describe the elements of normal psychology and social psychology.
6. Observe the principles of practice of medicine in hospital and community setting.

b. Skills

At the end of the course, the studnet should be able to make use of:

1. Principles of practice of medicine in hospital and community settings and familiarization with elementary nursing practices.
2. Art of **communication** with patients including history taking and medico-social work.

Teaching of community medicine, should be both theoretical as well as **practical.** The practical aspects of the training programme should include visits to the health establishements and to the community where health intervention programmes are in operation.

In order to inculcate in the minds of the students the basic concepts of community medicine to be introduced in this phase of training, it is suggested that the detailed curriculum drawn should include at least 30 hours of lectures, demonstrations, seminars, etc. together with at least 15 visits of two hours each.

PARA CLINICAL SUBJECTS OF PHASE II

5. COMMUNITY MEDICINE

i. Goal

The broad goal of the teaching of undergraduate students in Community Medicine is to prepare them to function as community and **first level physicians** in accordance with the institutional goals.

ii. Objectives

a. Knowledge

At the end of the course, the student should be able to:

1. Describe the health care delivery system including rehabilitation of the disabled in the country.
2. Describe the National Health Programmes with particular emphasis on maternal and child health programmes, family welfare planning and population control.
3. List epidemiological methods and describe their application to communicable and non-communicable diseases in the community or hospital situation.
4. Apply biostatistical methods and techniques;
5. Outline the demographic pattern of the country and appreciate the roles of the individual family, community and socio-cultural milieu in health and disease.
6. Describe the health information systems.

7. Enunciate the principles and components of primary health care and the national health policies to achieve the goal of 'Health for All'.
8. Identify the environmental and occupational hazards and their control.
9. Describe the importance of water and sanitation in human health.
10. To understand the principles of health economics, health administration, health education in relation to community.

b. Skills

All the end of the course, the student should be able to:

1. Use edidemiology as a scientific tool to make rational decisions relevant to community and individual patient intervention.
2. Collect, analyse, interpret and present simple community and hospital based data.
3. Diagnose and manage common health problems and emergencies at the individual, family and community levels keeping in mind the existing health care resources and in the context of the prevailing socio-cultural beliefs.
4. Diagnose and manage maternal and child health problems and advise a couple and the community on the family planning methods available in the context of the national priorities.
5. Diagnose and manage common nutritional problems at the individual and community level.
6. Plan, implement and evaluate a health education programme with the skill to use simple audio-visual aids.
7. Interact with other members of the health care team and participate in the organisation of health care services and implementations of national health programmes.

c. Integration

Develop capabilities of synthesis between cause of illness in the environment or community health and respond with leadership qualities to institute remedial measures for this.

CLINICAL SUBJECTS OF PHASE II AND PHASE III

FAMILY WELFARE PLANNING

Training in family welfare planning shall be emphasized in all the three phases and during internship as per guidelines.

The need for family welfare planning, organization of family welfare planning services, health eduction in relation to FP; nutrition psychological needs of mother, the child and the family and demography and vital statistics should be the major areas.

COMMUNITY MEDICINE

The teaching and training of community medicine will continue during the first two semesters of phase III (clinical phase). The goals, objectives and skills to be acquired by the students has already been outlined in phase II (paraclinical phase).

Internship

* Community medicine .... 2 months
* At community health centre/dist hospital
* At taluk hospital
* At primary health centre
* **Village attachment of at least one week to understand issues of community health along with ASHA and subcentre.**

Note: Learning/teaching contents of community medicine during various phases should be known to the students and methods of learning and teaching should be explained to them, besides methods of evaluation. Participatory learning should be the goal.

NATIONAL FAMILY HEALTH SURVEY-4 (NFHS-4)—2015-16

INDIA FACT SHEET

Introduction

The National Family Health Survey 2015–16 (NFHS-4), the fourth in the NFHS series, provides information on population, health and nutrition for India and each State/Union Territory. NFHS-4, for the first time, **provides district-level estimates** for many **important indicators**.

The contents of previous round of NFHS are generally retained and additional components are added from one round to another. In this round, information on malaria prevention, migration in the context of HIV, abortion, violence during pregnancy, etc. have been added. The scope of clinical, anthropometric, and biochemical testing (CAB) or Biomarker component has been expanded to include measurement of blood pressure and blood glucose levels. NFHS-4 sample has been designed to **provide district** and **higher** level estimates of various indicators covered in the survey. However, estimates of indicators of sexual behaviour, husband's background and woman's work, HIV/AIDS knowledge, attitudes and behaviour, and domestic violence will be available at **state and national level only**.

As in the earlier rounds, the Ministry of Health and Family Welfare, Government of India designated International Institute for Population Sciences, Mumbai as the nodal agency to conduct NFHS-4. The main objective of each successive round of the NFHS has been to provide essential data on health and family welfare and emerging issues in this area. NFHS-4 data will be useful in setting benchmarks and examining the progress in health sector the country has made over time. Besides providing evidence for the effectiveness of the ongoing programmes, the data from NFHS-4 help in identifying need for new programmes with area specific focus.

Four Survey Schedules—Household, Woman's, Man's and Biomarker-were canvassed in local language using Computer Assisted Personal Interviewing (CAPI). In the household schedule, information was collected on all usual members of the household and visitors who stayed in the household the previous night as well as socio-economic characteristics of the household, water and sanitation, health insurance, number of deaths in the household in the three years preceding the survey, etc. was canvassed in the Woman's schedule. The Man's schedule covered the man's characteristics, marriage, his number of children, contraception, fertility preferences, nutrition, sexual behaviour, attitudes towards gender roles, HIV/AIDS, etc. The biomarker schedule covered measurements of **height, weight** and **haemoglobin** levels for children; measurements of height, weight, haemoglobin levels, blood pressure, and random blood glucose level for women aged 15–49 years and men aged 15–54 years. In addition, women and men were requested to provide a few drops of blood from a finger prick for laboratory testing for HIV.

This fact sheet provides information on key indicators and trends for India. The figures of NFHS-4 and that of earlier rounds may not be strictly comparable due differences in sample size and NFHS-4 will be a benchmark for future surveys. NFHS-4 fieldwork for India was conducted from 20 January 2015 to 4 December 2016 by 14 Field Agencies and gathered information from 601,506 households, 699,686 women, and 103,525 men. Fact sheets for each State/UT and District of India are also available separately.

Table 1.1: India-Key Indicators on health and nutrition

Indicators	NFHS-4 (2015–16)			NFHS-3 (2005–06)
	Urban	Rural	Total	Total
Population and household Profile				
1. Population (female) age 6 years and above who ever attended school (%)	80.6	63.0	68.8	58.3
2. Population below age 15 years (%)	24.9	30.5	28.6	34.9
3. Sex ratio of the total population (females per 1,000 males)	956	1,009	991	1,000
4. Sex ratio at birth for children born in the last five years (females per 1,000 males)	899	927	919	914
5. Children under age 5 years whose birth was registered (%)	88.8	76.1	79.7	41.2
6. Households with electricity (%)	97.5	83.2	88.2	67.9
7. Households with an improved drinking-water source[1] (%)	91.1	89.3	89.9	87.6
8. Households with using improved sanitation facility[2] (%)	90.3	36.7	48.4	29.1
9. Households using clean fuel for cooking[3] (%)	80.6	24.0	43.8	25.5
10. Households using iodized salt (%)	96.5	91.4	93.1	76.1
11. Households with any usual member covered by a health scheme or health insurance (%)	28.2	29.0	28.7	4.8
Characteristics of Adult (age 15–49)				
12. Women who are literate (%)	81.4	61.5	68.4	55.1
13. Men who are iterate (%)	90.8	82.6	85.7	78.1
14. Women with 10 or more years of schooling (%)	51.5	27.3	35.7	22.3
Marriage and Fertility				
15. Women age 20–24 years married before age 18 years (%)	17.5	31.5	26.8	47.4
16. Men age 25–29 years married before age 21 years (%)	14.1	24.4	20.3	32.3
17. Total fertility rate (children per woman)	1.8	2.4	2.2	2.7
18. Women age 15–19 years who were already mothers or pregnant at the time of the survey (%)	5.0	9.2	7.9	16.0

(Contd...)

Table 1.1: India-Key Indicators on health and nutrition *(Contd...)*

Indicators	NFHS-4 (2015–16)			NFHS-3 (2005–06)
	Urban	Rural	Total	Total
Infant and Child Mortality Rates (per 1,000 live birts)				
19. Infant mortality rate (IMR)	29	46	41	57
20. Under-five mortality rate (U5MR)	34	56	50	74
Current use of family planning method (currently married women age 15–49 years)				
21. Any method[4] (%)	57.2	51.7	53.5	56.3
22. Any modern method[4] (%)	51.3	46.0	47.8	48.5
23. Female sterilization (%)	35.7	36.1	36.0	37.3
24. Male sterilization (%)	0.3	0.3	0.3	1.0
25. IUD/PPIUD (%)	2.4	1.1	1.5	1.7
26. Pill (%)	3.5	4.3	4.1	3.1
27. Condom (%)	9.0	3.9	5.6	5.2
Unmet Need for Family Planning (Currently married women age 15–49 years)[5]				
28. Total unmet need (%)	12.1	13.2	12.9	13.9
29. Unmet need for spacing (%)	5.1	5.9	5.7	6.1
Quality of Family Planning Services				
30. Health worker ever talked to female non-users about family planning (%)	18.6	17.2	17.7	10.1
31. Current users ever told about side effects of current method[6] (%)	50.1	45.0	46.5	34.4

[1] Piped water in dwelling/yard/plot, public tap/standpipe, tube well or borehole, protected dug well, protected spring, rainwater, community RO plant.

[2] Flush to piped sewer system, flush to septic tank, flush to pit latrine, ventilated improved pit (VIP)/biogas latrine, pit latrine with slab, twin pit/composting toilet, which is not shared with any other household.

[3] Electricity, LPG/natural gas, biogas.

[4] Includes other methods that are not shown separately.

[5] Unmet need for family planning refers to fecund women who are not using contraception but who wish to postpone the next birth (spacing) **or stop** childbearing altogether (limiting). Specifically, women and considered to have unmet need for spacing if they are:

• At risk of becoming pregnant, not using contraception, and either do not want to become pregnant within the next two years, or are unsure if or when they want to become pregnant.

• Pregnant with a mistimed pregnancy

• Postpartum amenorrheic for up to two years following a mistimed birth and not using contraception.

Women are considered to have unmet need for limiting if they are:
- At risk of becoming pregnant, not using contraception, and want no (more) children.
- Pregnant with an unwanted pregnancy.
- Postpartum amenorrheic for up to two years following an unwanted birth and not using contraction.

  Women who are classified as infecund have no unmet need because they are not at risk of becoming pregnant. Unmet need for family planning is the sum of unmet need for spacing plus unmet need for limiting.

[6] Based on current users of female sterilization, IUD/PPIUD, injectables and pill who started using that method in the past 5 years.

Table 1.1: India-Key Indicators on Health and Nutrition *(Contd...)*				
	NFHS-4 (2015–16)			NFHS-3 (2005–06)
Indicators	Urban	Rural	Total	Total
Maternal and Child Health				
Maternity care (for last birth in the 5 years before the survey)				
32. Mothers who had antenatal check-up in the first trimester (%)	69.1	54.2	58.6	43.9
33. Mothers who had at least 4 antenatal care visits (%)	66.4	44.8	51.2	37.0
34. Mothers whose last birth was protected against neonatal tetanus[7] (%)	89.9	88.6	89.0	76.0
35. Mothers who consumed iron folic acid for 100 days or more when they were pregnant (%)	40.8	25.9	30.3	15.2
36. Mothers who had full antenatal care[8] (%)	31.1	16.7	21.0	11.6
37. Registered pregnancies for which the mother received Mother and Child Protection (MCP) card (%)	87.7	90.0	89.3	na
38. Mothers who received postnatal care from a doctor/nurse/LHV/ ANM/midwife/other health personnel within 2 days of delivery (%)	71.7	58.5	62.4	34.6
39. Mothers who received financial assistance under Janani Suraksha Yojana (JSY) for births delivered in an institution (%)	21.4	43.8	36.4	na

(Contd...)

Table 1.1: India-Key Indicators on Health and Nutrition *(Contd...)*

Indicators	NFHS-4 (2015–16)			NFHS-3 (2005–06)
	Urban	*Rural*	*Total*	*Total*
40. Average out of pocket expenditure per delivery in public health facility (Rs.)	3,913	2,947	**3,198**	na
41. Children born at home who were taken to a health facility for check-up within 24 hours of birth (%)	3.2	2.4	2.5	0.3
42. Children who received a health check after birth from a doctor/nurse/ LHV/ANM/midwife/other health personnel within 2 days of birth (%)	27.2	23.0	24.3	na
Delivery Care (for births in the 5 years before the survey)				
43. Institutional births (%)	88.7	75.1	78.9	38.7
44. Institutional births in public facility (%)	46.2	54.1	52.1	18.0
45. Home delivery conducted by skilled health personnel (out of total deliveries) (%)	3.0	4.9	4.3	8.2
46. Births assisted by a doctor/nurse/ LHV/ANM/ other health personnel(%)	90.0	78.0	81.4	46.6
47. Births delivered by caesarean section (%)	28.3	12.9	17.2	8.5
48. Births in a private health facility delivered by caesarean section (%)	44.8	37.8	40.9	27.7
49. Births in a public health facility delivered by caesarean section (%)	19.9	9.3	11.9	15.2
Child Immunizations and Vitamin A Supplementation				
50. Children age 12–23 months fully immunized (BCG, measles, and 3 doses each of polio and DPT) (%)	63.9	61.3	62.0	43.5
51. Children age 12–23 months who have received BCG (%)	93.2	91.4	91.9	78.2
52. Children age 12–23 months who have received 3 doses of polio vaccine (%)	73.4	72.6	72.8	78.2
53. Children age 12–23 months who have received 3 doses of DPT vaccine (%)	80.2	77.7	78.4	55.3
54. Children age 12–23 months who have received measles vaccine (%)	83.2	80.3	81.1	58.8

(Contd...)

Table 1.1: India-Key Indicators on Health and Nutrition *(Contd...)*

Indicators	NFHS-4 (2015–16)			NFHS-3 (2005–06)
	Urban	*Rural*	*Total*	*Total*
55. Children age 12–23 months who have received 3 doses of hepatitis B vaccine (%)	63.3	62.5	62.8	na
56. Children age 9–59 months who received a vitamin A dose in last 6 months (%)	62.9	59.1	60.2	16.5
57. Children age 12–23 months who received most of the vaccinations in public health facility (%)	82.1	94.2	90.7	82.0
58. Children age 12–23 months who received most of the vaccinations in private health facility (%)	16.7	3.4	7.2	10.5
Treatment of Childhood Diseases (children under age 5 years)				
59. Prevalence of diarrhoea (reported) in the last 2 weeks preceding the survey (%)	8.2	9.6	9.2	9.0
60. Children with diarrhoea in the last 2 weeks who received oral rehydration salts (ORS) (%)	58.5	47.9	50.6	26.0
61. Children with diarrhoea in the last 2 weeks who received zinc (%)	23.7	19.1	20.3	na
62. Children with diarrhoea in the last 2 weeks taken to a health facility (%)	74.1	65.8	67.9	61.3
63. Prevalence of symptoms of acute respiratory infection (ARI) in the last 2 weeks preceding the survey (%)	2.3	2.9	2.7	5.8
64. Children with fever or symptoms of ARI in the last 2 weeks preceding the survey taken to a health facility (%)	80.0	70.8	73.2	69.6
Child Feeding Practices and Nutritional Status of Children				
65. Children under age 3 years breastfed within one hour of birth[9] (%)	42.8	41.1	41.6	23.4
66. Children under age 6 months exclusively breastfed[10] (%)	52.1	56.0	54.9	46.4
67. Children age 6–8 months receiving solid or semi-solid food and breastmilk (%)	50.1	39.9	42.7	52.6
68. Breastfeeding children age 6–23 months receiving an adequate diet[10, 11] (%)	10.1	8.2	8.7	na

(Contd...)

Table 1.1: India-Key Indicators on Health and Nutrition *(Contd...)*

Indicators	NFHS-4 (2015–16)			NFHS-3 (2005–06)
	Urban	Rural	Total	Total
69. Non-breastfeeding children age 6–23 months receiving an adequate diet[10, 11] (%)	16.9	12.7	14.3	na
70. Total children age 6–23 months receiving an adequate diet[10, 11] (%)	11.6	8.8	9.6	na
71. Children under 5 years who are stunted (height-for-age)[12] (%)	31.0	41.2	38.4	48.0
72. Children under 5 years who are wasted (weight-for-height)[12] (%)	20.0	21.5	21.0	19.8
73. Children under 5 years who are severely wasted (weight-for-height)[13] (%)	7.5	7.4	7.5	6.4
74. Children under 5 years who are underweight (weight-for-age)[12] (%)	29.1	38.3	35.9	42.5

[7] Includes mothers with two injections during the pregnancy of her last birth, or two or more injections (the last within 3 years of the last live birth), or three or more injections (the last within 5 years of the last birth), or four or more injections (the last within 10 years of the last live birth), or five or more injections at any time prior to the last birth.

[8] Full antenatal care is at least four antenatal visits, at least one tetanus toxoid (TT) injection and took iron folic acid tablets or syrup for 100 or more days.

[9] Based on the last child born in the 5 years before the survey.

[10] Based on the youngest child living with the mother.

[11] Breastfed children receiving 4 or more food groups and a minimum meal frequency, non-breastfed children fed with a minimum of 3 Infant and Young Child Feeding Practices (fed with other milk or milk products at least twice a day, a minimum meal frequency that is receiving solid or semi-solid food at least twice a day for breastfed infants 6–8 months and at least three times a day for breastfed children 9–23 months, and solid or semi-solid foods from at least four food groups not including the milk or milk products food group).

[12] Below 2 standard deviations, based on the WHO standard.

[13] Below 3 standard deviations, based on the WHO standard.

Table 1.1: India-Key Indicators on Health and Nutrition

Indicators	NFHS-4 (2015–16)			NFHS-3 (2005–06)
	Urban	Rural	Total	Total
Nutritional Status of Adults (age 15–49 years)				
75. Women whose Body Mass Index (BMI) is below normal (BMI < 18.5 kg/m^2)14 (%)	15.5	26.7	22.9	35.5

(Contd...)

Table 1.1: India-Key Indicators on Health and Nutrition *(Contd...)*

Indicators	NFHS-4 (2015–16) Urban	Rural	Total	NFHS-3 (2005–06) Total
76. Men whose Body Mass Index (BMI) is below normal (BMI < 18.5 kg/m^2) (%)	15.3	23.0	20.2	34.2
77. Women who are overweight or obese (BMI ≥ 25.0 kg/m^2)[14] (%)	31.3	15.0	20.7	12.6
78. Men who are overweight or obese (BMI ≥ 25.0 kg/m^2) (%)	26.3	14.3	18.6	9.3
Anaemia among Children and Adults[15]				
79. Children age 6–59 months who are anaemic (<11.0 g/dl) (%)	55.9	59.4	58.4	69.4
80. Non-pregnant women age 15–49 years who are anaemic (<12.0 g/dl) (%)	50.9	54.3	53.1	55.2
81. Pregnant women age 15–49 years who are anaemic (<11.0 g/dl) (%)	45.7	52.1	50.3	57.9
82. All women age 15–49 years who are anaemic (%)	50.8	54.2	53.0	55.3
83. Men age 15–49 years who are anaemic (<13.0 g/dl) (%)	18.4	25.2	22.7	24.2
Blood Sugar Level among Adults (age 15–49 years)[16]				
Women				
84. Blood sugar level - high (>140 mg/dl) (%)	6.9	5.2	5.8 na	8.6
85. Blood sugar level - very high (>160 mg/dl) (%)	3.6	2.3	2.8	na
Men				
86. Blood sugar level - high (>140 mg/dl) (%)	8.8	7.4	8.0 11.9	na
87. Blood sugar level - very high (>160 mg/dl) (%) hypertension among adults (age 15–49 years)	4.4	3.5	3.9	na
Women				
88. Slightly above normal (systolic 140–159 mm of Hg and/or diastolic 90–99 mm of Hg) (%)	7.3	6.5	6.7	na
89. Moderately high (systolic 160–179 mm of Hg and/or diastolic 100–109 mm of Hg) (%)	1.6	1.3	1.4 8.8	na
90. Very high (systolic[3] 180 mm of Hg and/or diastolic [3] 110 mm of Hg) (%)	0.7	0.7	0.7	na

(Contd...)

Table 1.1: India-Key Indicators on Health and Nutrition *(Contd...)*

Indicators	NFHS-4 (2015–16) Urban	Rural	Total	NFHS-3 (2005–06) Total
Men				
91. Slightly above normal (systolic 140–159 mm of Hg and/or diastolic 90–99 mm of Hg) (%)	11.4	9.8	10.4	na
92. Moderately high (systolic 160–179 mm of Hg and/or diastolic 100–109 mm of Hg) (%)	2.7	2.0	2.3 13.6	na
93. Very high (systolic^3 180 mm of Hg and/or diastolic^3 110 mm of Hg) (%)	1.0	0.8	0.9	na
Women Age 15–49 Years Who Have Ever Undergone Examinations of:				
94. Cervix (%)	25.3	20.7	22.3	na
95. Breast (%)	11.7	8.8	9.8	na
96. Oral cavity (%)	15.6	10.7	12.4	na
Knowledge of HIV/AIDS among Adults (age 15–49 years)				
97. Women who have comprehensive knowledge[17] of HIV/AIDS (%)	28.1	16.9	20.9	17.3
98. Men who have comprehensive knowledge[17] of HIV/AIDS (%)	37.4	29.3	32.3	33.0
99. Women who know that consistent condom use can reduce the chances of getting HIV/AIDS (%)	67.0	41.1	54.9	36.3
100. Men who know that consistent condom use can reduce the chances of getting HIV/AIDS (%)	83.4	73.9	77.4	70.0
Women's Empowerment and Gender Based Violence (age 15–49 years)				
101. Currently married women who usually participate in household decisions (%)	85.8	83.0	84.0	76.5
102. Women who worked in the last 12 months who were paid in cash (%)	23.2	25.4	24.6	28.6
103. Ever-married women who have ever experienced spousal violence (%)	23.6	31.4	28.8	37.2
104. Ever-married women who have experienced violence during any pregnancy (%)	2.9	3.5	3.3	na
105. Women owning a house and/or land (alone or jointly with others) (%)	35.2	40.1	38.4	na

(Contd...)

Table 1.1: India-Key Indicators on Health and Nutrition *(Contd...)*

Indicators	NFHS-4 (2015–16) Urban	Rural	Total	NFHS-3 (2005–06) Total
106. Women having a bank or savings account that they themselves use (%)	61.0	45.5	53.0	15.1
107. Women having a mobile phone that they themselves use (%)	61.8	36.9	45.9	na
108. Women age 15–24 years who use hygienic methods of protection during their menstrual period[18] (%)	77.5	48.2	57.6	na
Tobacco Use and Alcohol Consumption among Adults (age 15–49 years)				
109. Women who use any kind of tobacco (%)	4.4	8.1	6.8	10.8
110. Men who use any kind of tobacco (%)	38.9	48.0	44.5	57.0
111. Women who consume alcohol (%)	0.7	1.5	1.2	2.2
112. Men who consume alcohol (%)	28.7	29.5	29.2	31.9
113. Women who tried to stop smoking or using tobacco in any other form during the past 12 months[19] (%)	33.0	28.2	29.3	na
114. Men who tried to stop smoking or using tobacco in any other form (during the past 12 months)[19] (%)	29.6	31.2	30.6	na

[14]Excludes pregnant women and women with a birth in the preceding 2 months.

[15]Haemoglobin in grams per decilitre (g/dl). Among children, prevalence is adjusted for altitude. Among adults, prevalence is adjusted for altitude and for smoking status.

[16]Random blood sugar measurement (including those under medication).

[17]Comprehensive knowledge means knowing that consistent use of condoms every time they have sex and having just one uninfected faithful sex partner can reduce the chance of getting HIV/AIDS, knowing that a healthy-looking person can have HIV/AIDS, and rejecting the two most common misconceptions about transmission or prevention of HIV/AIDS.

[18]Locally prepared napkins, sanitary napkins and tampons are considered as hygienic methods of protection.

[19]Based on those who currently smoke or use tobacco

Note: NFHS4 essentially gathered the information from households/families. NFHS4 data of respective state/districts is also available. Students can be given learning excercises for presentation of these data by diagrams, analysis and interpretation of data for actions at various levels. Live epidemiological excercises can be developed from these data. NFHS data uses cut of levels for various parameters, which can be used as reference standards.

MAJOR HEALTH PROBLEMS IN INDIA IN 2016 (Table 1.2)

India bears almost one-fifth burden of the world's disease.

i. The burden of most infectious and associated diseases reduced in India from 1990 to 2016. The disease burden due to communicable, maternal and nutritional diseases contributed 32.7% of DALYs losses down from 61% in 1990, while Noncommunicable diseases contributed 55.4% up from 30% in 1990, and injuries contributed to 12% of DALYs losses in the year 2016 up from 9% in 1990. (Fig. 1.1).

ii. **Problem:** Over the last 26 years the burden of most infectious and associated diseases has declined in better of states but still high in weaker States of Uttrakhand, Bihar, Chhatisgarh, UP, MP and North East State groups. The share of NCDs in total burden of disease has increased in well to do states due to unhealthy life styles. Punjab is the capital of ischaemic heart disease in India.

iii. **Therapy:** Therapy is to adopt healthier life styles by community and increase public health spending from a woeful low of 1.15% of GDP to at least 2.5% of GDP as stated in National health Policy 2017.

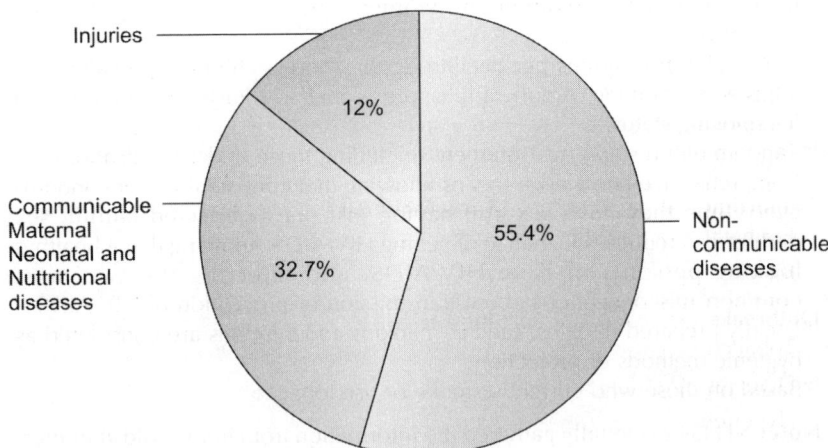

Fig. 1.1: Disease burden (measured in DALYs Losses) by Major disease groups in India 2016.*

Source: ICMR, PHFI, and IHME India: Health of the Nation's States—The India State Level Disease Burden Initiative 2016.

Table 1.2: Major Health Problems in India

Total population in 2015	1311 million
Total fertility rate	2.2
Crude birth rate	20.8
Sex ratio census 2011	940
Female illiteracy 2011	31.6%
People below poverty line 2012	21.9%
Human development index rank 2015	131

Disease Burden

India's share in Global disease burden 2015	19%
India's share in global incidence of TB Do	27%
Burden of TB in India 2014 (prevalence)	2.5 million
Leprosy-new cases per year	1.27 lakh
HIV burden-people living with HIV/AIDS	2.11 million
STI/reproductive tract infections-episodes per year	30 million
Malaria incidence per year 2016	1 million
Filaria cases	1.2 million
Iodine deficiency disorders	71 million
Any mental morbidity	10.6%
Anaemia in pregnancy	50%
Maternal mortality ratio 2015	174
Infant mortality rate 2016	34
Under five mortality rate	45
Low birth weight babies	28%
Underweight children below 5 years	35.7%
Proportion of deaths due to NCDs	60%

Proportion of Deaths due to CCDs, Maternal

Perinatal and nutritional	28%
Injuries	12%

Outbreaks—Dengue, Chikungunia, HINI, JE   **Frequent**

Tobacco use in adults	28.6%
Diabetes in adults	Women 8.6% Men 11.6%
Hypertension in adults	Women 8.8% men 13.6%
Overweight and obese	Women 20.7% men 18.6%
Coronary heart disease	1.6% to 7.4% in rural and 6.5 to 13.2% in urban areas
Chronic obstructive resp. diseases	3.3 to 5.4%

Thus major disease burden is due to noncommunicable disease followed by communicable diseases and nutritional deficiency in children, adolescent and pregnant women.

Major Causes and Determinants of Health Problems in India

- Rapid population growth and unplanned urbanization.
- Poverty and ignorance.
- Deteriorating environments—water, soil and air pollution.
- Unhealthy life styles.
- Wide spread nutritional deficiencies.
- Nutrition excess in well to do.
- Road Traffic accidents/injuries.
- Weak public health system.
- Illiteracy—lack of information and poor utilization of available services.
- Migration of population, growing international trade, tourism and rapid population movement.
- Illicit drugs/substance abuse including tobacco and alcohol use.
- Natural disasters.
- Antimicrobial resistance-irrational drug use.
- Insecticide resistance.
- Heredity and genetics.

HOUSEHOLD/FAMILY-BASIC UNIT OF LEARNING IN COMMUNITY MEDICINE

The household information consists of:

Household No	House No	Family type	Nuclear/Joint
Religion	Caste	Source of drinking water	Storage practices
Monthly income	Above poverty line	Below poverty line	Type of latrine
Type of house	Katcha-pucca-semi-pucca	Ownership of house	Own-Rented
Number of rooms	Separate kitchen	Type of fuel used	
Assets	TV-Radio	Other assets	Motor vehicle, tractor
Breeding places of mosquitoes and flies	Land holding	Cattle wealth	Garbage and waste water dispossal

Household (HH) Surveys

HH surveys are conducted at the village or ward level by a team of ASHA, AWW and trained TBA. The main purpose is to determine health care needs of population, resource mapping and also to assess as how social determinants of health influence the health of households such as drinking water, sanitary latrines, employment and access to other health requirements (Table 1.3).

Table 1.3: Individual Information-at Household Level											
1	2	3	4	5	6	7	8	9	10	11	12
Name of head of household	Name of members of household	Age in years DOB	Sex	Relation to head of household	Marital status	Occupation and literacy	Immunization status of children	Illness in last one month	disability if any	Marriages pregnancy births deaths in the last year	Health care utilization and expenditure

Household information and household survey data are used for community health needs assessment and to prepare village health action plan, to determine work load and setting targets by the health workers themselves. This also ensures community participation in planning and monitoring health activities.

The households and family are places where child care and maternal care practices, gender discrimination and health care seeking behaviours are learned and find their support from community. Hence household and families should be supported by health system by regular contacts/visits of health team. Households and families be linked with dynamic health system for continuity of care.

Improving family household practices that can help to promote child survival and safe-motherhood are:

i. Exclusive breastfeeding for first 6 months of life.

ii. Complementary feeding-feeding children energy and nutrient rich complementary food while coutinuing to breastfeed for at least 2 years-can reduce mortality by 10%.

iii. Micronutrient supplementation—improving the intake of vitamin A through diet or supplements can reduce mortality in young children.

iv. Hygiene—hand washing and safe disposal of excreta can reduce incidence of diarrhoea by 35%.

v. Immunization—measles and others.

vi. Psychological care and development—provide early psychosocial stimulation by mother child interaction.

vii. Feeding and fluids to sick children.

viii. Care seeking for sick children

ix. Antenatal care—tetanus toxoid, safe delivery, care during post-partum and lactation period.

NITI Aayog

The National Institution for Transforming India, also called NITI Aayog, was formed via a resolution of the Union Cabinet on January 1, 2015. NITI Aayog is the premier policy 'Think Tank' of the Government of India, providing both directional and policy inputs. While designing strategic and long term policies and programmes for the Government of India, NITI Aayog also provides relevant technical advice to the Centre and States.

The Government of India, in keeping with its reform agenda, constituted the NITI Aayog to replace the Planning Commission instituted in 1950. This was done in order to better serve the needs and aspirations of the people of India. An important evolutionary change from the past, NITI Aayog acts as the quintessential platform of the Government of India to bring States to act together in national interest, and thereby fosters cooperative federalism.

At the core of NITI Aayog's creation are two hubs—**Team India Hub** and the **Knowledge and Innovation Hub.** The Team India Hub leads the engagement of states with the central government, while the Knowledge and Innovation Hub builds NITI's think-tank capabilities. These hubs reflect the two key tasks of the Aayog.

NITI Aayog is also developing itself as a State of the Art Resource Centre, with the necessary resources, knowledge and skills, that will enable it to act with speed, promote research and innovation, provide strategic policy vision for the government, and deal with contingent issues.

After the end of 12th plan on March 2017, India would have a 15 years vision document to realize long terms goals. People's aspirations and priorities as determined by every "Gram Sabha and equivalent urban bodies" of the country shall be the basis of planning process. It would be a "Planning by the people, for the people and with the people".

2

Application of Social and Behavioural Sciences in Health and Disease Management

Disability Adjusted Life Years (DALYs): Developed by WHO and World Bank, DALY is widely used to measure the global disease burden. One DALY can be interpreted as equalling one year of healthy life lost.

For example, a person who is expected to live up to 70 years but dies prematurely due to stroke at 65 years, has lost 5 DALYs. DALYs combine (a) losses from premature deaths which is defined as the difference between actual age at death and life expectancy at that age in a low mortality population and (b) loss of healthy life resulting from disability. Percentage of DALYs losses in India in 2016:

- Communicable diseases 32.7%

- Noncommunicable diseases 55.4%

- Injuries 12%

National Health Policy 2017 states to establish regular tracking of Disability Adjusted Life Years Index as a measure of burden of disease and its trends by major categories by 2020.

3

Determinants of Health—Health Policy and Goals

NATIONAL HEALTH POLICY 2017

The National Health Policy of 1983 and the National Health Policy of 2002 have served well in guiding the approach for health sector in five-year plans. Now 15 years after the last health policy, the situation has changed in five major ways. First, the health priorities are changing. There is growing burden of noncommunicable diseases and some infectious diseases. The second important change is the emergence of a robust health care industry. The third change is growing incidence of catastrophic health expenditure due to health care costs, leading to poverty. Fourth, a rising economic growth enables enhanced fiscal capacity. Fifth important change is Sustainable Development Goals set by United Nations. Therefore, new health policy responsive to these contextual changes is required. NHP 2017 builds on the progress made since the last NHP of 2002 and 1983. A policy is as good as its implementation. Health is a state responsibility. States are to play key role in implementation of the stated health policy.

1. NATIONAL HEALTH POLICY-2017—GOAL AND OBJECTIVES
GOAL
The attainment of the highest possible level of "Health and well being for all at all ages" and achieve "Sustainable Development Goals" of United Nations by 2030.

Objectives
- Progressively achieve **Universal Health Coverage**
  a. Assuring availability of free comprehensive primary health care services, for all aspects of reproductive, maternal, child

and adolescent health and for most prevalent communicable and noncommunicable diseases and occupational diseases in population.
  b. Improved access to affordable, quality secondary and tertiary health care through combination of public and private providers.
  c. To achieve reduction in out of pocket expenditure and catastrophic health expenditure.
  • Reinforcing trust in public health care system.
  • Align the growth of private care sector with public health goals.

2. NATIONAL HEALTH POLICY (NHP) 2017—SPECIFIC OBJECTIVES

The specific objective of NHP are in line with Sustainable Development Goals of UNs.

A. Health Status and Programme Impact by 2025
  • Increase life expectancy at birth from 67.5 to 70 years.
  • Reduction of total fertility rate to 2.1.
  • Reduce under five mortality rate to 23.
  • Reduce MMR from current level to 100.
  • Reduce infant mortality rate to 28.
  • Reduce neonatal mortality rate to 16 and "still birth rate to single digit".

Reduction of Disease Burden (Prevalence and Incidence)
  • HIV-achieve global target of 90 : 90 : 90.
  • Achieve and maintain elimination of leprosy, kala-azar and lymphatic filariasis by 2017 and 2018.
  • TB: Achieve cure rate of over 85% in new sputum positive patients, reduce incidence and reach elimination by 2025.
  • To reduce prevalence of blindness to 0.25%.
  • To reduce pre-mature mortality from cardiovascular diseases, cancer, diabetes and chronic respiratory diseases, by 25%

B. Health Systems Performance
  • Increase utilization of public health facilities by 50% from current levels of 30%.
  • Achieve antenatal care coverage above 90%.
  • Skilled attendance at birth above 90%.
  • Coverage of fully immunized infants above 90%.

- Meet family planning needs above 90%.
- 80% of known hypertensives and diabetics at household level maintain controlled disease status.

Health Related Cross Sectoral Goals

- Reduce prevalence of tobacco use by 15% by 2020 and 30% by 2025.
- Reduce prevalence of stunting by 40% in under five children.
- Access to safe water and sanitation to all by 2020.
- Reduction of occupational injuries by half from current levels of 334 per lakh.

C. Health System Strengthening—Health Finances

- Increase health expenditure by government as percentage of GDP from existing 1.15 to 2.5% by 2025.
- Decrease in proportion of households facing catastrophic health expenditure from the current levels by 25% by 2025.
- Increase state health sector spending to more than 8% of their budget.

D. Health infrastructure and Human Resources

Paramedicals and doctors as per IPHS or national norms in priority districts.

E. Health Management Information System

Ensure district level electronic data base and strengthen surveillance system.

3. POLICY THRUST AREAS

Raising public health expenditure to 2.5% of GDP in time bound manner.

Preventive and promotive health: "Health in all" as complement to "Health for all" the policy identifies **seven** priority areas to address social **determinants** of **health** through intersectoral cordination.

Seven Priority Areas

- The Swachh Bharat Abhiyan (Reduction of water, excreta and vector borne diseases).
- Balanced healthy diets and regular excercises.
- Addressing tobacco, alcohol and substance abuse.

- Yatri suraksha-preventing deaths due to rail, road traffic accidents.
- Nirbhay-Nari-Action against gender violence.
- Reduced stress and improved safety at work place.
- Reduce indoor and outdoor air pollution.

Organization of public health care delivery: The policy proposes seven **key policy shifts** in organizing health care services:

i. In primary health care—from selective care to assured **comprehensive Primary Health Care** with linkages to referral hospitals for continuity of services.

ii. In secondary and tertiary care—from an **input oriented** budget line financing to an **output based** strategic purchasing from public/private hospitals.

iii. In public hospitals—from **user fees** and **cost recovery** to **assured free drugs, diagnostic** and **emergency services** to all.

iv. In infrastructure and human resource development—from **normative approach** to **targeted approach** to reach under-serviced areas.

v. In Urban Health—from **token interventions** to on-scale **assured interventions,** to organize Primary Health Care delivery and referral support for urban poor. Collaboration with other sectors to address wider determinants of urban health is advocated.

vi. In National Health Programmes—**Integration with health systems** for programme effectiveness and in turn contributions to strengthening of health systems for efficiency.

vii. In AYUSH services—from **stand-alone to** a three dimensional **mainstreaming** (co-location of AYUSH, availability of standard medicines and protocols and YOGA).

Strategies of Care

a. Free primary health care provision by **public sector**.

b. **Strategic purchase** of secondary care, hospitalization and tertiary care services from both public and from Non Government sector to fill critical gap would be the **main strategy**.

c. Mainstreaming of different health systems (AYUSH).

Spectrum of Services

a. Free primary care services and continuity of care

- Upgradation of existing subcentres and reorientation of PHCs to "Health and Wellness Centers" to provide package of

comprehensive preventive, promotive, curative and rehabilitative services.
- Linking every family/household to primary health care facility package anywhere in the country (health care to every family).
- Two way systemic linkages between primary, secondary and tertiary services to ensure continuity of care.
- *Screening*: Early detection and response to early childhood development delays and disability .
- Adolescent and sexual health eduction.
- Behaviour change with respect to tobacco, alcohol and drugs and physical inactivity.
- Counseling for primary prevention and secondary pervention for common chronic illness—both communicable and non-communicable diseases.
- School health, occupational health, tribal health to cover 100 million tribal population, urban health, and control of zoonotic diseases.

b. *Secondary care services*

- To provide most of the secondary care at district and sub-district level hospitals.
- Two beds per thousand population distributed in such a way that it is accessible within golden hour rule, by having efficient emergency transport system. Ten categories of specialist services/skills be available at district and 4–5 at sub-district hospital level.
- *Reorienting public hospital*: Public hospitals would provide universal access to progressively wide array of free drugs, diagnostics and emergency services of high quality.
- *Closing infrastructure and human resources/skill gaps*: The policy follows road map of 12th five year plan for managing human resources for health as per Indian Public Health Standards/National norms.
- *Urban Health Care*: Establish Urban Health Centres, Urban Community Health Centres for Urban poor/slum areas for comprehensive urban primary health services. Give primacy to local bodies.

4. NATIONAL HEALTH PROGRAMMES (NHPs)

- **Example:** RMNCH +A, Communicable and Noncommunicable diseases, mental health, Trauma centres and occupational health. Integration of NHPs with health systems for effectiveness and in turn strengthening of health systems for efficiency.

- *Population stabilization*: Improve static services for family planning and **increase men participation** from less than 1% currently to 30% (sterilizations).

5–6. WOMEN'S HEALTH AND GENDER MAINSTREAMING

Enhanced provision for reproductive morbidities and health needs of women beyond reproductive age group (40+), orientation of staff to gender sensitive and women friendly services and provide free services with dignity to victims of gender violence.

7. SUPPORTIVE SUPERVISION

Supporting innovative measures of supportive supervision in more vulnerable districts.

8. EMERGENCY CARE AND DISASTER PREPAREDNESS

Better response to disasters both man made and natural. Life support ambulances and Trauma management centres one for 30 lakh in urban and one for 10 lakh in rural areas.

9. MAINSTREAMING POTENTIALS OF AYUSH

Bridge courses for AYUSH to prepare workforce of mid-level care providers at the level of subcentre.

10. TERTIARY HEALTH CARE SERVICES

The policy affirms that tertiary care services are best organized along line of regional, zonal and apex referral centres. Govt should set up new Medical Collages, Nursing Institutions and AIIMS like institutions. Purchase select tertiary health care services from Non Government sector hospitals to assist the poor.

11. HUMAN RESOURCES IN HEALTH

- Medical and paramedical eduction be integrated with the service delivery system so that students learn in the real environment and not just in confines of medical schools.
- Medical eduction—strengthening existing medical colleges and converting district hospitals to new medical colleges to increase number of doctors and specialists.
- Revision of curriculum of UGs and PGs.
- Develop a cadre of mid—level service providers.
- Nursing eduction—improve regulations.

- Para medical skills—training courses and curriculum for super speciality paramedical care.
- Public health management cadre—creation of public health management cadre in all states.
- Human resource governance and leadership: Human-resource management and continuing medical and nursing eduction and policies on recruitment, selection, promotion, posting, and transfer and leadership skills for good governance.

12. FINANCING OF HEALTH SERVICES

- Allocation of major proportion of up to 67% or more of resources to primary health care followed by secondary and tertiary care. Public health account in health has been set up.
- Strategic purchasing of secondary and tertiary health care to fill the critical gaps in services.

13. COLLABORATION WITH NON GOVERNMENT SECTOR/ ENGAGEMENT WITH PRIVATE SECTOR

The policy advocates positive and proactive engagement with private sector for critical gap filling, towards achieving national public health goals.

Areas: Outsourcing of training of teachers, as corporate social responsibility (CSR), primary health care services, engaging private hospital for skill development in collaboration with national council for skill development, mental health care programme, disaster management, strategic purchasing of secondary and tertiary care from private sector, diagnostic services, ambulance services, referral services, immunizations, disease surveillance and notification, and various national health programmes and other areas like health information system and outsourcing of diagnostic and tertiary care etc. Private sector should be supported for skill upgradation and rational drug use and use of standard treatment protocols as also "Make in India".

14. REGULATORY FRAMEWORK

Regulation of professional education—six professional councils, clinical establishments, food safety, drug regulation, medical devices, vaccines safety and medical technology, etc.

15. ESSENTIAL DRUGS AND DIAGNOSTICS

Promoting generic drugs and technologies besides well developed procurement system of drugs.

16. HEALTH RESEARCH

Increase investment in health research in the areas of health system and services research, medical product innovation, fundamental research, and translational research, etc.

17. GOVERNANCE

Role of centre and state governments and their accountability; directorates to be strengthened by HR (Human Resources) policies, those from public health management cadre must hold senior positions in public health. Involve PRIs and local bodies, encourage community monitoring system.

18. IMPLEMENTATION FRAMEWORK

Put in place the implementation framework. A policy is only as good as its implementation.

4

Population Stabilization and Declining Child Sex Ratio

TOTAL FERTILITY RATES (TFR) NEARING TARGET

Government of India has categorized states as per the TFR level into very high focus states (more than or equal to 3.0 TFR) high focus states (TFR More than 2.1 and less than 3.0) and non high focus states (TFR less than or equal to 2.1) for adopting different strategies. Further 146 priority districts have been identified in high focus and very high focus states in the country for intensive efforts. Target is to bring TFR of 2.1 or less by 2030 in all the states. Current level of TFR was 2.2 in the year 2015 close to the target of 2.1 and achievable by 2025 in all the states (Table 4.1).

FAMILY PLANING SCENARIO

Data of NFHS-4, and DLHS-4 and AHS are being used to describe current family planning situation in India. Nationwide small family norm is widely accepted and the general awareness of contraception is almost universal (over 98%). Contraceptive use rate among married women (couples) (aged 15–49 years) was 53.5%. Female sterilization was the most popular method of contraception (36%),

Table 4.1: Total fertility rates (TFR) in various states 2014	
TFR of 2.1 or less (Non high focus states)	24 states and UTs of India
TFR of 2.2 to 3.0 (High focus states)	10 states—Haryana 2.2, Gujarat 2.3, Arunachal 2.3, Assam 2.3, Dadar and Nagar Haveli 2.4 Chhattisgarh 2.6, Jharkhand 2.8, Rajasthan 2.8, MP. 2.8, Meghalaya 2.9
TFR above 3.0 (Very high focus states)	2 States—Bihar 3.2 and UP 3.2

followed by condoms (5.6%), oral pills (4.1%), IUCD (1.5%) male sterilization 0.3% and traditional methods were being used by 6% of couples (Fig. 4.1).

The proximate determinates of fertility rate like age of marriage and age at first child birth (which are societal preferences) are also showing improvement at national level. However men participation in contraception is low and spacing methods need to be improved aggressively on voluntary basis; through social marketing and behavior change communication. Use rate of oral contraceptive is on the increase while IUCD and condom use rates are almost static at 1.5% and 5.6% respectively.

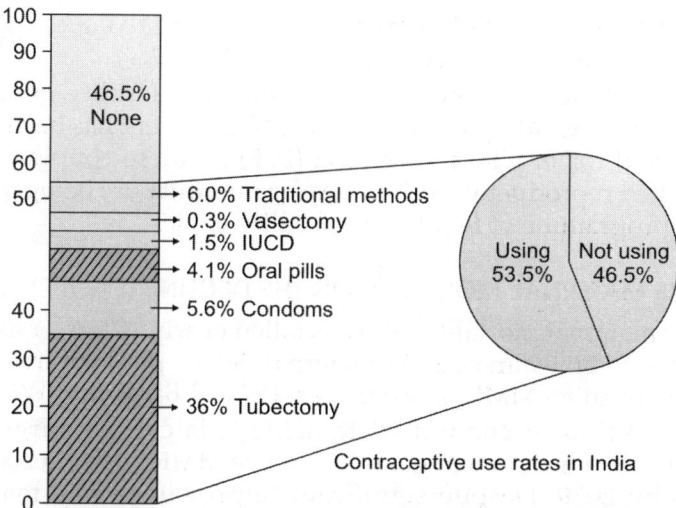

Fig. 4.1: Contraceptive use rates in India 2015–16

India's 'Vision FP 2020'

India's global commitment made at London summit 2012 to achieve the goals of:

i. Providing family planning services to 48 million additional women and sustain coverage of 100 million users till 2020.

ii. Aversion of 23.9 million births

Aversion of 1 million infant deaths

Aversion of 42000 maternal deaths by 2020

iii. Reaching couple protection rate of 63.7%.

iv. To bring the family planning programme back to centre stage to reduce the unmet needs of contraception and to avert thousands of maternal and infant deaths due to unwanted pregnancies.

Unmet Needs in Family Planing

Total unmet needs for family planning was 12.9%, while unmet need for spacing being 5.7% and 7.2% for terminal methods.

New Initiatives

- Injectable contraceptives (DMPA) have been introduced into family planning programme under ANTARA programme (one injection every three months interval).
- POP (progestrone oral pill) and centchroman (CHHAYA).
- Delivery of contraceptives by ASHAs at doorstep.
- Home based pregnancy testing kits (NISCHAY).
- As per WHO data the prevalence rate of infertility in various countries including India is about 10–15% There has been rising demand for *in vitro* fertilization (IVF) by these couples, hence assisted reproductive techniques for infertility are being used in the programme at regulated infertility clinics.

INDIA'S MATERNAL MORTALITY ON THE DECLINE (Fig. 4.2)

India's maternal mortality ratio has fallen nearly 70% over the past 25 years, to an estimated 174 maternal deaths per lakh live births in 2015, from an MMR of 556 in 1990 (World Bank, and WHO).

India has also committed to achieve latest UN targets for sustainable development goals to achieve MMR 70 per 100000 live births by 2030. Despite significant improvements in maternal

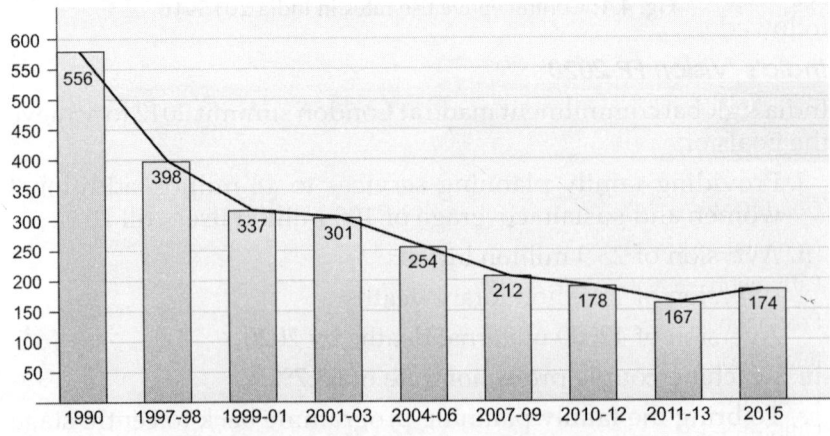

Fig. 4.2: Trends of maternal mortality ratio in India

mortality an estimated 45000 mothers continue to die every year due to causes related to pregnancy, childbirth and the post-partum period. The major medical causes of these deaths are haemorrhages, sepsis, unsafe abortions, hypertensive disorders, obstructed labour, and 'other' causes including anaemia.

New initiatives: Besides promotion of institutional deliveries, prevention of post-partum haemorrhages (PPH) (loss of more than 500–1000 ml blood within first 2 hours of birth) through community based advance distribution of **3 Misoprostol tablets of 200 mg each** by ASHAs/ANMs has been launched for >20% home delivery districts. Five National Skill Labs "Daksh" at Delhi and NCR with support from maternal health division, Govt of India and Liverpool School of Tropical Medicine have been established along with 30 stand alone skill labs in different states to improve quality of training in RMNCH + A services.

ii. Direct Benefits Transfer under JSY

Now JSY incentive money in being transferred to the account of pregnant women linked with Aadhar.

iii. Pradhan Mantri Surakshit Matritva Abhiyan (PMSMA)

A new boost has been given to reduce maternal mortality through PMSMA popularly referred to as "I pledge 9" (scheme to provide free health check ups to pregnant women). That was announced by Prime Minister during his Man Ki Baat on June 2015. On fixed day, i.e. 9th of every month, quality antenatal care universally to all pregnant women is being provided with active participation of public and private sectors. These services are in addition to routine services, high risk pregnancies are identified and referred to and followed up regularly.

CURRENT STATUS OF CHILD MORTALITY IN INDIA AND SUSTAINABLE DEVELOPMENT GOALS BY 2030		
Child health indicator	*Current status*	*SDG Goal 2030*
Neonatal mortality rate	26	Less than 10
Early neonatal mortality rate	20	–
Post-neonatal mortality rate	13	–
Infant mortality rate (2016)	34	–
Under five mortality rate	45	25
Stillbirth rate (2011)	22	<10

Major causes of infant mortality in India in 2012 (WHO) were perinatal conditions 46%, respiratory infections 22%, diarrhoeal diseases 10%, Other infections and parasitic diseases 8%, and congenital abnormalities 3.1%.

New Initiatives

1. **"MAA**—Mother's Absolute Affection" Programme to promote universal exclusive breastfeeding has been initiated in August 2016—a one year intensive awareness drive on breast feeding promotion.
2. **Newer vaccines**—Rotavirus and Pneumococcal conjugate vaccines have been introduced to prevent diarrhoea and pneumonia morbidity and mortality.

5

Reproductive and Child Health—Policy and Programmes in India

LIFE-SAVING COMMODITIES IN RMNCH + A PROGRAMME

With a strong focus on the reproductive, maternal, newborn and child health (RMNCH) 'Continuum of Care', the UN Commission identified and endorsed an initial list of 13 overlooked life-saving commodities that, if more widely accessed and properly used, could save the lives of more than 6 million women and children.

RMNCH continuum of care	Commodity	Usage
Reproductive health	• Female condoms	Family planning/contraception
	• Implants	Family planning/contraception
	• Emergency contraception	Family planning/contraception
Maternal Health	• Oxytocin	Post-partum haemorrhage
	• Misoprostol	Post-partum haemorrhage
	• Magnesium sulfate	Eclampsia and severe pre-eclampsia toxemia of pregnancy
Newborn Health	• Injectable antibiotics	Newborn sepsis
	• Antenatal corticosteroid (ANCS)	Respiratory distress syndrome for preterm babies
	• Chlorhexidine	Newborn cord care
	• Resuscitation equipment	Newborn asphyxia
Child Health	• Amoxicillin	Pneumonia
	• Oral rehydration salts (ORS)	Diarrhoea
	• Zinc	Diarrhoea

Criteria

The commission looked at three criteria to identify these commodities:

1. *High-impact, effective commodities*: In general, high-impact commodities are those commodities that effectively address avoidable causes of premature death and disease among children under five years old and women during pregnancy and childbirth.
2. *Inadequate funding*: Selected commodities are not funded by existing mechanisms such as The Global Fund to fight AIDS, tuberculosis and malaria, Global Alliance for Vaccines and Immunisation (GAVI), Scaling-up Nutrition (SUN) and UNAID.
3. *Untapped potential*: Innovation and rapid scale-up in product development and market shaping (including potential for price reduction and improved stability of supply) arising from the work of a UN Commission could rapidly improve access to the selected commodities.

Expected Impact

The Commission estimated that an ambitious scaling up of these 13 commodities over five years would cost less than US$ 2.6 billion and would cumulatively save over 6 million lives including 230,000 maternal deaths averted through increased access to family planning.

Achieving these goals would save an extra 1.8 million child deaths a year, reducing the estimated 7.1 million deaths in 2010 to 5.3 million. Likewise, the estimated 287,000 maternal deaths in 2010 would be reduced to 213,000 by increased access to maternal health and family planning commodities.

IMNCI IN INDIA

IMNCI STRATEGIES

i. Improving case management skills of providers by training.
ii. Improving overall health systems and inter-sectoral coordination.
iii. Improving family and community health practices. First two components are facility based and the third one most weakest is community based.

Promoting Health Behaviours/Practices at Community and Household Level such as

- Initiation of breast feeding within an hour after birth.
- Exclusive breast feeding for 6 months.
- Adequate complementary feeding.
- Vitamin A supplementation.
- Immunizatin against pertussis, measles, Hib, Pneumococcal Conjugate Vaccine and Rotavirus vaccine under UIP.
- Use safe drinking water and sanitary latrines.
- Hand washing with soap and water.
- Reduce household air pollution, HIV prevention.
- Continue feeding during illness.
- Oral rehydration therapy.
- Early care seeking and compliance of care at home.

Ensure counselling of care givers during home visits on recognition of illness, on feeding, growth monitoring and overall health promotion, besides involvement of mothers and community. This component is being ignored in IMNCI and it needs to be strengthened and promoted aggressively.

INTEGRATED ACTION PLAN FOR PNEUMONIA AND DIARRHOEA

Pneumonia and diarrhoea together are responsible for 27% of deaths in under five children in India. Significant proportion of these deaths are amenable to prevention at community level. Therefore an integrated Global Action Plan for pneumonia and Diarrhoea (GAPPD) was Launched in 2013 with the aim of ending preventable deaths from pneumonia and diarrhoea by 2025.

SPECIFIC OBJECTIVES

- To reduce deaths from pneumonia to fewer than 3 per 1000 live births in under five children.
- To reduce deaths from diarrhoea to less than 1 per 1000 live births in children under five years of age.
- Reduce malnutrition by 40%.

As an adaptation of GAPPD, the Government of India along with WHO and UNICEF in September 2014 developed an integrated action plan for pneumonia and diarrhoea (IAPPD). The plan is focusing on four states—Uttar Pradesh, Bihar, Rajasthan, Madhya Pradesh which account for more than half of under five deaths[7].

Proven interventions to tackle pneumonia and diarrhoea exist. Children are dying because services are provided piecemeal and those most at risk are not being reached. Use rate of effective interventions remain too low. For instance only in 41.6% of births breast-feeding is initiated within an hour, 54.9% are exclusively breastfed up to 6 months and ORS use rate is low at 50.6% and 73.6% of children with ARI are taken to health facility. The problem of pneumonia and diarrhoea must be addressed in an integrated manner as envisaged under IMNCI strategy. Coverage must be enhanced to achieve the objectives.

Integrated Strategies

1. Protect Children

- By establishing **best health practices** from birth onward.
- Exclusive breastfeeding for 6 months and continued breast-feeding.
- With adequate complementary feeding and complementary breastfeeding up to 2 years of age or more.
- Vitamin A supplementation reduces the onset and severity of diarrhoea and pneumonia.

2. Prevent Children from Becoming Ill by

- *Use of vaccines*: Against pertussis, measles, Hib, PCV and Rotavirus–achieve 80% coverage. *Streptococcus pneumoniae* and *Haemophilus influenzae* type B are most common causes of childhood pneumonia.
- *Handwashig* with soap and water.
- Safe drinking water and sanitation-universal access.
- Reduce household air pollution by ventilation and improved fuel/stoves.
- HIV prevention.
- Cotrimoxazole prophylaxis for HIV infected and exposed children.

3. *Treating Children who are Ill from Pneumonia and Diarrhoea*

- Improve care seeking and referrals.
- Standard case management practices at the health facility and community level.
- Supplies—low osmolarity ORS, Zinc, antibiotics and oxygen. (Life saving commodities).
- Continue feeding (including breastfeeding).

The progress towards implementation will be measured by district score cards.

Applied Nutrition Programmes/Interventions

MOTHER'S ABSOLUTE AFFECTION (MAA) PROGRAMME FOR PROMOTION OF BREASTFEEDING 2016

Breastfeeding within an hour of birth could prevent 20% of neonatal mortality, the substantial increase in institutional deliveries (over 80%) following launch of JSY and Janani Shishu Suraksha Karyakram has provided an excellent opportunity for ensuring early initiation of breastfeeding. However, only 41.6% of mothers initiate breastfeeding within one hour of birth in spite of the fact the about 80% deliver in institutions. Further 54.9% babies are exclusively breastfed during first six months and 42.7% of children between 6 and 8 months received solid/semisolid food and breastmilk. There is need to improve these rates and practices at community and institutional level. MAA (Mother's Absolute Affection) Programme supports promotion, protection of breast feeding practices by intensified communication activities at all the levels of health care.

Exclusive breastfeeding for first six months and appropriate infant and young child feeding practices are being promoted in convergence with Ministry of Women and Child Development. Ministry of health and family welfare launched "MAA—Mother's Absolute Affection" Programme in August 2016 for improving breastfeeding practices:

a. Initiate breastfeeding within one hour of birth.

b. Universal exclusive breastfeeding up to 6 months and

c. Complementary breastfeeding up to 2 years of age throuɟh mass media and capacity building of health care providers in health facilities as well as in communities. MAA is primarily a communication strategy to promote breast feeding.

PROBLEM OF LOW BIRTH WEIGHT BABIES

In India 28% of babies born have low birth weight (less than 2500 g)

LBW babies fall under two categories:
  a. Small for gestational age, i.e. they are full term babies and have IUGR.
  b. Preterm babies born before 37th weeks of gestation.

  Low-birth weight is a predominant cause of infant mortality. Causes of low birth weight babies in India are:
  i. Adolescent and maternal under nutrition (Anaemia).
  ii. Early marriages and teenage pregnancies.
  iii. Less spacing between births.
  iv. High birth orders
  v. Lack of antenatal care service or poor utilization of antenatal care, besides inadequate diet and IFA consumption.

PREVENTION AND CONTROL OF SOIL TRANSMITTED HELMINTHS (NTD)

NATIONAL DEWORMING DAY (NDD)

Ministry of Health and Family Welfare had adopted a single day strategy called National Deworming Day (NDD) in 2015 to combat Soil Transmitted Helminths (STH) infections in children. During NDD a single dose of Albendazole 400 mg is administered to the children of 1–19 years age by school teachers and anganwadi workers. In the year February 2016 NDD reached to 250 million children in 34 States/UTs.

Ministry of Health and Family Welfare has also established STH (Soil Transmitted Helminths) surveillance mechanism across the country under the aegis of National Centre for Disease Control. Based on STH prevalence data, MOH and FW conducted 2nd round of deworming in 27 states and UTs where STH prevalence is high. About 150 million children were covered in august 2016. This programme along with Biweekly iron and folic acid to children 6–59 months and weekly iron and folic acid tablets to children between 5 and 10 years will improve the nutritional status of young children along with promotion of sanitary latrines and eduction on nutrition and personal hygiene. Soil transmitted helminths—*See* Chapter 7, page 276. STH are neglected tropical diseases (NTDs).

Potassium Bromate Banned

- A harmful additive cancer causing chemical—potassium bromate has been banned in bread by Ministry of Health in India. The chemical was being used to enhance the texture of the bread. The FSSA (Food Safety and Standard Act of India) has approved and published standards for food additives and ingredients.

Haryana Demonstration Project on Wheat Flour Fortification to Improve Iron, Folate, and Vitamin B_{12} Status

The burden of iron deficiency anemia and neural tube defects (NTDs) is high in India. Iron and folic acid supplementation programs have not been very successful in addressing these concerns adequately. Some states in India have already initiated wheat flour fortification to address micronutrient deficiencies. Average NTDs prevalence in India is about 41 per 10,000 live births.

The Haryana government has committed to introduce wheat flour fortification as a pilot program to demonstrate the health impact of fortified wheat flour. Prior to the state-wide introduction of fortification, this pilot program will be launched in the rural areas of two blocks of Ambala (Naraingarh and Barara) in 3 phases over a five-year period. The purpose of the Haryana Demonstration Project is to assess the feasibility, sustainability, and health impact of fortifying wheat flour using India's existing open market and government systems in Ambala District.

Fortification is adding vitamins and minerals to foods to prevent nutritional deficiencies. The nutrients regularly used in grain fortification prevent diseases, strengthen immune systems, and improve productivity and cognitive development. Fortification is successful because it makes frequently eaten foods more nutritious without changing the food habits. Wheat flour fortification has been introduced and proven successful in many countries to address NTDs and iron deficiency anemia.

Vitamins and minerals often used in wheat flour fortification and their role in health include:

- Iron, folic acid, vitamin B_{12} help prevent nutritional anemia which improves productivity, maternal health, and cognit.ve development.
- Folic acid (vitamin B_9) reduces the risk of neural tube birth defects
- Vitamin B_{12} maintains functions of the brain and nervous system.

NATIONAL NUTRITION MISSION (NNM) 2017-20

NNM has been set up in the year 2017 GOAL:

I. To reduce stunting, wasting and low birth weight by 2% per annum and anaemia among children, women and adolescent girls by 3% per annum.

II. Reduce stunting from 38.4% in 2016 to 25% by 2022.

The mission will supervise, monitor and fix targets for the existing anti-malnutrition plans to steer them in right direction. These schemes include—ICDS, JSY, mid-day-meal and National Food Security Mission. The NNM will bring in convergence of different ministries apart from technology based real time monitoring growth of children as well as check the pilferage of food/ration provided at Anganwadis. Services delivered by ANMs, AWWs, ASHAs will be monitored and SMS alert sent to parents on progress of child health and nutrition for early actions.

Environmental Health

AIR POLLUTION

About 90% of people are breathing poor quality of air. Air pollution is a global public health emergency. Over 60% of people in India use unprocessed biomass fuel for cooking which leads to indoor air pollution. NFHS4 data indicates that only 43.8% of households in India use clean fuel. To combat climate change 197 countries agreed to phase out Hydrofluorocarbons (HCF) use by 85% by 2045 as per Kigall Amendment to Montreal Protocol, and freezing production and consumption of HCF.

WHO Air Quality Guidelines

Particulate matter: Annual mean values of 20 $\mu g/m^3$ (for PM10) and 10 $\mu g/m^3$ (for PM2.5).

8

Epidemiology and its Applications in Prevention and Control of Diseases and Epidemics

Table 8.1: Association between ice cream consumption and development of vomiting and diarrhoea in the year 2015 in marriage party

		Cases	Controlls	Total	Attack rate
Consumption of ice cream	Yes	80	20	100	80%
	No	10	30	40	25%
	Total	90	50	140	64%

$$\text{Relative risk or risk ratio} = \frac{\text{Attack rate in exposed}}{\text{Attack rate in unexposed}} = \frac{80}{25} = 3.2$$

ODDS ratio = $(80 : 10) \div (20 : 30)$

$$= \frac{80}{20} \frac{30}{10} = 12$$

Proportion of cases exposed = 80/90 = 89%
Proportion of controls exposed = 20/50 = 40%
Population attributable risk percent = 64–25/64 = 61%

Attributable risk or risk difference: It is attack rate in exposed minus attack rate in unexposed = 80–25 = 55% is risk attributable to ice-cream consumption (Table 8.1).

When comparing the cases of vomiting and diarrhoea with controls there was high proportion of case patients (80/90 = 89%) who consumed ice cream as compared to controls (20/50 = 40%).

The risk ratio is calculated as the ratio of the attack rates or risks in exposed/attack rates or risks in unexposed, i.e. 80 divided by 25 which equals 3.2. This means those who consumed ice-cream were 3.2 times more likely to develop vomiting and diarrhoea than those who did not consume ice cream. Hence there is strong association with consumption of ice cream and occurrence of diarrhoea and vomiting. When the attack rate for the exposed group is the same as the attack rate for the unexposed group, the risk ratio or relative risk is equal to 1.0, which denotes no association with exposure. ODDS ratio of 12 further confirms strong association with the exposure.

COHORT STUDY

Risk difference or attributable risk = 120 − 40 = 80

The incidence of 80/1000 infant deaths was attributable to low birth weight in this study.

Percentage attributable risk in the population

This is incidence of infant deaths in total population (−) incidence of infant deaths in births with adequate weight divided by incidence of infant deaths in total population.

$$= \frac{67 \quad 40}{67} = \frac{27}{67} \quad 100 = 40\%$$

This means 40% of total infant mortality could be prevented in the population if the risk factor of low birth weight is eliminated in the community.

EPIDEMIC CURVES

Epidemic referes to an increase, often sudden, in number of cases of a disease above what is normally expected in that population in that area.

Epidemic Patterns

Epidemics can be classified according to their manner of spread in population:
1. **Common source—Point, continuous** and **intermmitent.**
2. **Propagated**
3. **Mixed**
4. **Others**

Epidemic curves are basic investigative tools as they provide wealth of information.
1. The epidemic curve shows magnitude of the epidemic over time as a simple, easily understood visual. It permits the investigator to distinguish epidemic from endemic disease.
2. The shape of epidemic curve may provide clues about the pattern of spread in the population, e.g. point, versus intermmitent source versus propagated.

3. The curve shows where you are in the course of the epidemic— still on the upswing, on the down slope, or after the epidemic has ended. This information forms the basis for predicting whether more or fewer cases will occur in the near future.

4. The curve can be used for **evaluation**, answering questions like how long did it take for the health department to identify a problem? Are intervention measures working?

5. **Outliers**—cases that donot fit into the body of curve may provide important clues.

6. If the disease and its incubation period are known, the epi curve can be used to deduce the **probable time of exposure** and help develop a questionaire focused on that time period.

Interpreting an Epidemic Curve (Figs 8.1a to c)

Shape: An epidemic curve that has a steep rise and a more gradual decline is characteristic of a **point source epidemic** in which persons are exposed to the same source over a relative brief period. In point source epidemic, all the cases occur within one incubation period. If the duration of exposure is prolonged, the epidemic is called a **Continuous Common Source Epidemic** and epidemic curve has a plateu instead of a peak.

• An intermittent common-source epidemic (in which exposure to the causative agent is sporadic over time) usually produces an irregularly jagged epidemic curve reflecting the intermittence and duration of exposure and the number of persons exposed.

• **In theory a propagated epidemic**—one spread from person to person with increasing number of cases in each generation–

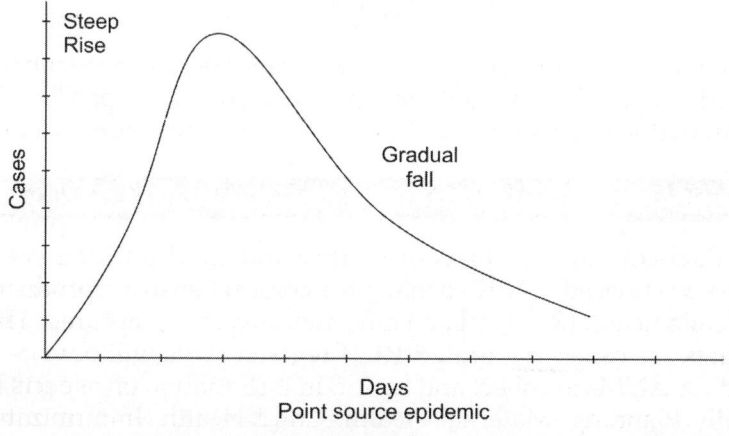

Point source epidemic

Fig. 8.1a

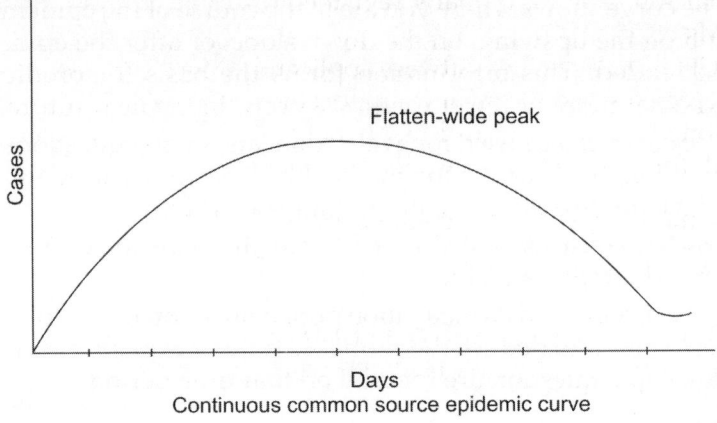

Fig. 8.1b

Continuous common source epidemic curve

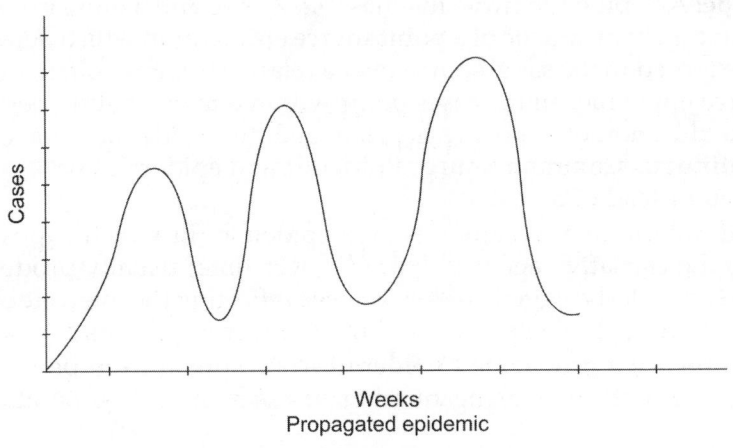

Fig. 8.1c

Propagated epidemic

should have a series of progressively taller peaks one incubation period apart, but in reality few produce this classic pattern. One can deduce likely period of exposure from the epidemic curve.

HEALTH MANAGEMENT INFORMATION SYSTEM (HMIS)

The data collection formats of mother and child tracking system have been revised in 2017 so that more comprehensive reproductive and child health (RCH) related information may be captured. These formats are called **integrated RCH register**. This will obviate the need for ANMs to collect and maintain information on aspects like Family Planning, Maternal Health, Child Health, Immunization, Mortality, etc. in multiple registers, often resulting in entering similar information in many registers, resulting in duplication of ANMs efforts.

RCH Portal is online software application based on the integrated RCH register to promote and support the RMNCH + A programme (lifelong tracking of individual beneficiary). The revised monthly HMIS for subcentre is as under:

Revised Monthly HMIS Format (Sub-Centre-SC) April 2017		
Sl. no.	*Data item*	*Numbers reported during the month*
PART A	REPRODUCTIVE AND CHILD HEALTH	
M1	Ante Natal Care (ANC) Services	
1.1	Total number of pregnant women registered for ANC	
1.1.1.	Out of the total ANC registered, number registered within 1st trimester (within 12 weeks)	
1.2	Tetanus Toxoid (TT) Immunisation to Pregnant Women (PW)	
1.2.1	Number of PW given TT1	
1.2.2	Number of PW given TT2	
1.2.3	Number of PW given TT Booster	
1.2.4	Number of PW given 180 iron folic acid (IFA) tablets	
1.2.5	Number of PW given 360 calcium tablets	
1.2.6	Number of PW given one albendazole tablet after the 1st trimester	
1.2.7	Number of PW received 4 or more ANC check ups	
1.2.8	Number of PW given ANC corticosteroids in preterm labour	
1.3	Pregnant Women (PW) with Hypertension (BP >140/90	
1.3.1	New cases of PW with hypertension detected	
1.3.1.a	Out of the new cases of PW with hypertension detected, cases managed at institution	
1.4	Pregnant Women (PW) with Anaemia	
1.4.1	Number of PW tested for Haemoglobin (Hb)	

(Contd...)

Revised Monthly HMIS Format (Sub-Centre-SC) April 2017 *(Contd...)*

Sl. no.	Data item	Numbers reported during the month
1.4.2	Number of PW having Hb level <11 (tested cases)	
1.4.3	Number of PW having Hb level <7 (tested cases)	
1.5	**Pregnant Women (PW) with Syphilis**	
1.5.1	Point of care (POC) tests conducted for syphilis	
1.5.1.a	Number of PW tested using POC test for syphilis	
1.5.1.b	Out of above, number of PW found sero-positive for syphilis	
M2	**Deliveries**	
2.1	**Deliveries conducted at home**	
2.1.1	**Number of home deliveries**	
2.1.1.a	Number of home deliveries attended by Skill Birth Attendant (SBA) (Doctor/Nurse/ANM)	
2.1.1.b	Number of home deliveries attended by Non SBA trained birth attendant (TBA)/Relatives/etc.	
2.1.2	Number of PW given tablet misoprostol during home delivery	
2.1.3	Number of newborns received 7 home based newborn care (HBNC) visits in case of home delivery	
2.2	Number of institutional deliveries conducted	
2.2.1	Out of total institutional deliveries number of women discharged within 48 hours of delivery	
2.2.2	Number of newborns received 6 HBNC vists after institutional delivery	
M3	**Pregnancy outcome and details of new-born**	
3.1	**Pregnancy outcome (in number)**	
3.1.1	**Live birts**	
3.1.1.a	Live birth—male	
3.1.1.b	Live birth—female	
3.1.2	Number of preterm newborns (<37 weeks of pregnancy)	

(Contd...)

(Contd...)

3.1.3	Stillbirth
3.2	Abortion (spontaneous)
3.3	**Details of Newborn Children**
3.3.1	Number of newborns weighed at birth
3.3.2	Number of newborns having weight less than 2.5 kg
3.3.3	Number of newborns breastfed within 1 hour of birth
M4	**Post Natal Care (PNC)**
4.1	Women receiving 1st postpartum checkup within 48 hours of home delivery
4.2	Women receiving 1st postpartum checkup between 48 hours and 14 days
4.3	Number of mothers provided full course of 180 IFA tablets after delivery
4.4	Number of mothers provided 360 calcium tablets after delivery
M5	**Family Planning**
5.1	Number of interval IUCD insertions (excluding PPIUCD and PAIUCD)
5.2	Number of postpartum (within 48 hours of delivery) IUCD insertions
5.3	Number of IUCD removals
5.4	Number of complications following IUCD insertion
5.5	Injectable Contraceptive-Antara Program-first dose
5.6	Injectable Contraceptive-Antara Program-second dose
5.7	Injectable Contraceptive-Antara Program-third dose
5.8	Injectable Contraceptive-Antara Program-fourth or more than fourth
5.9	Number of combined oral pill cycles distributed
5.10	Number of condom pieces distributed
5.11	Number of centchroman (weekly) pills strips distributed
5.12	Number of emergency contraceptive pills (ECP) given

(Contd...)

Revised Monthly HMIS Format (Sub-Centre-SC) April 2017 *(Contd...)*

Sl. no.	Data item	Numbers reported during the month
5.13	Number of pregnancy test kits (PTK) used	
5.10	**Quality in sterilization services**	
5.10.1	Complications following male sterilization	
5.10.2	Complications following female sterilization	
M6	**CHILD IMMUNISATION**	
6.1	**Number of Infants 0 to 11 months old who received:**	
6.1.1	Vitamin K (Birth Dose)	
6.1.2	BCG OPV at birth	
6.1.3	DPT1, 2, 3	
6.1.4	Child immunisation—pentavalent 1, 2, 3	
6.1.5	Child immunisation—OPV1, 2, 3	
6.1.6	Child immunisation—hepatitis-B1, 2, 3	
6.1.7	Inactivated injectable polio vaccine (FIPV1)	
6.1.8	Inactivated injectable polio vaccine (FIPV2)	
6.1.9	Rotavirus 1, 2, 3	
6.2	Number of children 9–11 months who received	
6.2.1	Child immunisation (9–11 months)—measles and rubella (MR)-1st Dose	
6.2.2	Child immunisation (9–11 months)—Measles 1st dose	
6.2.3	Child immunisation (9–11 months)—JE 1st dose	
6.2.4	**Number of chidren aged between 9 and 11 months fully immunized (BCG + DPT 123/pentavalent 123 + OPV123 + Measles**	
6.2.4a	Children aged between 9 and 11 months fully immunized—Male	
6.2.4b	Children aged between 9 and 11 months fully immunized—Female	
6.3	Children given following vaccination after 12 months	
6.3.1	Child immunisation—measles and rubella (MR)-1st dose	
6.3.2	Child immunisation—measles-1st dose	
6.3.3	Child immunisation-JE 1st dose	

(Contd...)

(Contd...)

6.4	**Number of Children more than 12 months who received**
6.4.1	Child immunisation—measles and Rubella (MR)—2nd Dose (16–24 months)
6.4.2	Child immunisation—measles—2nd dose (More than 16 months)
6.4.3	Child immunisation—DPT—1st Booster
6.4.4	Child immunisation—OPV booster
6.4.5	Child immunisation—measles, mumps, rubella (MMR) vaccine
6.4.6	Number of children more than 16 months of age who received Japanese encephalitis (JE) vaccine
6.5	**Number of Children more than 23 Months who received**
6.5.1	Child immunisation—Typhoid
6.5.2	Children more than 5 years received DPT (2nd Booster)
6.5.3	Children more than 10 years received TT10
6.5.4	Children more than 16 years received TT16
6.6	**Adverse Event Following Immunisation (AEFI)**
6.6.1	Number of cases of AEFI—abscess
6.6.2	Number of cases of AEFI—deaths
6.6.3	Number of immunisation session where ASHAs were present
6.8	**Children received Vitamin A Doses between 9 Months and 5 years**
6.8.1	Child immunisation—Vitamin A dose 1
6.8.2	Child immunisation—Vitamin A dose 5
6.8.3	Child immunisation—Vitamin A dose 9
6.9	Number of children (6–59 months) provided 8–10 doses (1 ml) of IFA syrup (Bi weekly)
6.10	Number of children (12–59 months) provided albendazole
6.11	Number of severely underweight children provided health checkup (0–5 yrs)
M7	**Number of cases of Childhood Diseases (0–5 years)**
7.1	Childhood Diseases—tuberculosis (TB)

(Contd...)

Revised Monthly HMIS Format (Sub-Centre-SC) April 2017 *(Contd...)*

Sl. no.	Data item	Numbers reported during the month
7.2	Childhood Diseases—acute flaccid paralysis (AFP)	
7.3	Childhood Diseases—measles	
7.4	Childhood Diseases—malaria	
7.5	Childhood Diseases—diarrhoea	
M8	**National Vector Borne Disease Control Programme (NVBDCP)**	
8.1	**Malaria**	
8.1.1	**Rapid Diagnostic Test (RDT)**	
8.1.1.a	RDT conducted for malaria	
8.1.1.b	Malaria (RDT)—*Plasmodium vivax test* positive	
8.1.1.c	Malaria (RDT)—*Plamodium falciparum* test positive	
Part B	**Health Facility Services**	
M9	**Patient Services**	
9.1	**Outpatient Department (Outpatients) by Disease/Health Condition**	
9.1.1	Outpatient—diabetes	
9.1.2	Outpatient—hypertension	
9.1.3	Outpatient—stroke (paralysis)	
9.1.4	Outpatient—acute heart diseases	
9.1.5	Outpatient—mental illness	
9.1.6	Outpatient—epilepsy	
9.1.7	Outpatient—ophthalmic related	
9.1.8	Outpatient—dental	
9.2	**Outpatient attendance (All)**	
9.2.1	Allopathic—outpatient attendance	
9.2.2	Ayush—outpatient attendance	
9.3	Number of Anganwadi centres/UPHCs reported to have conducted Village Health and Nutrition Day (VHND)/ Urban Health and Nutrition Day (UHND)/Outreach/Special Outreach	
M10	**Laboratory Testing**	
10.1	**Hb Tests Conducted**	
10.1.1	Number of Hb tests conducted	

(Contd...)

(Contd...)

10.1.2	Out of the total number of Hb tests done, Number having Hb <7 mg	
10.2	Human Immuno-deficiency Virus (HIV) tests conducted	
10.2.1	**Antenatal Cases tested for HIV**	
10.2.1.a	Number tested for HIV (numbers screened)	
10.2.1.b	Out of the numbers screened, number Tested for HIV Integrated Counselling and Testing Centre (ICTC) tested cases)	
10.2.1.c	Number Positive for HIV (numbers confirmed positive at ICTCs)	
M11	**Stock Related Data**	
11.1	**Drugs**	
11.1.1	Last date of supply of essential drugs	
11.1.2	**Items**	**Adeqate/Inadequate**
11.1.2.a	IFA tablets	
11.1.2.b	IFA syrup with dispenser	
11.1.2.c	Vit A syrup	
11.1.2.d	ORS packets	
11.1.2.e	Zinc tablets	
11.1.2.f	Inj magnesium sulfate	
11.1.2.g	Inj oxytocin	
11.1.2.h	Misoprostol tablets	
11.1.2.i	Antibiotics	
11.1.2.j	Availability of drugs for common ailments, e.g. PCM, anti-allergic drugs, etc.	
11.1.2.k	IFA tablets (blue)	
11.1.2.l	Tab. albendazole	
11.2	**Vaccine**	
11.2.1	Last date of supply of essential vaccines	
11.2.2	**Items**	**Adeqate/Inadequate**
11.2.2.a	TT	
11.2.2.b	BCG	
11.2.2.c	Hepatitis	
11.2.2.d	OPV	

(Contd...)

Revised Monthly HMIS Format (Sub-Centre-SC) April 2017 *(Contd...)*

Sl. no.	*Data item*	*Numbers reported during the month*
11.2.2.e	DPT	
11.2.2.f	Measles	
11.2.2.g	Vitamin A	
11.3	**Contraceptive**	
11.3.1	Last date of supply of essential contraceptive	
11.3.2	**Items**	**Adeqate/Inadequate**
11.3.2.a	IUCD	
11.3.2.b	Combined oral pills (in cycles)	
11.3.2.c	Condom (in pieces)	
11.3.2.d	Injectable contraceptive MPA (vials)	
Part C M12	**Mortality Details** **Details of Deaths Reported with Probable Causes**	
12.1	Infant deaths within 24 hrs (1 to 23 hrs) of birth	
12.2	**Infant Deaths up to 4 weeks (1 to 28 days) due to**	
12.2.1	Infant deaths up to 4 weeks due to Sepsis	
12.2.2	Infant deaths up to 4 weeks due to Asphyxia	
12.2.3	Infant deaths up to 4 weeks due to other causes	
12.3	**Infant Deaths between 1 month (more than 28 days) and less than 12 months due to**	
12.3.1	Number of infant deaths (1–12 months) due to pneumonia	
12.3.2	Number of infant deaths (1–12 months) due to diarrhoea	
12.3.3	Number of infant deaths (1–12 months) due to fever related	
12.3.4	Number of infant deaths (1–12 months) due to measles	
12.3.5	Number of infant deaths (1–12 months) due to other causes	

(Contd...)

(Contd...)

12.4	**Child Deaths between 1 year and less than 5 years due to**
12.4.1	Number of child deaths (1–5 years) due to pneumonia
12.4.2	Number of child deaths (1–5 years) due to diarrhoea
12.4.3	Number of child deaths (1–5 years) due to fever related
12.4.4	Number of child deaths (1–5 years) due to measles
12.4.5	Number of child deaths (1–5 years) due to other causes
12.5	**Maternal Deaths (15 to 49 yrs.) due to**
12.5.1	Number of maternal deaths due to bleeding
12.5.2	Number of maternal deaths due to high fever
12.5.3	Number of maternal deaths due to abortion
12.5.4	Number of maternal deaths due to obstructed/prolonged labour
12.5.5	Number of maternal deaths due to severe hypertesnion/fits
12.5.6	Number of maternal deaths due to other causes (including causes not known)
12.6	**Other Deaths (except Infant, Child and Maternal Deaths) 5 years and above**
12.3.1	Number of adolescent/adult deaths due to diarrhoea diseases
12.3.2	Number of adolescent/adult deaths due to tuberculosis
12.6.3	Number of adolescent/adult deaths due to respiratory diseases including infections (other than TB)
12.6.4	Number of adolescent/adult deaths due to other fever related
12.6.5	Number of adolescent/adult deaths due to HIV/AIDS
12.6.6	Number of adolescent/adult deaths due to heart disease/hypertension related

(Contd...)

Revised Monthly HMIS Format (Sub-Centre-SC) April 2017 *(Contd...)*

Sl. no.	Data item	Numbers reported during the month
12.6.7	Number of adolescent/adult deaths due to cancer	
12.6.8	Number of adolescent/adult deaths due to neurological disease including strokes	
12.6.9	Number of adolescent/adult deaths due to accidents/burn cases	
12.6.10	Number of adolescent/adult deaths due to suicide	
12.6.11	Number of adolescent/adult deaths due to animal bites and sting	
12.6.12	Number of adolescent/adult deaths due to known acute disease	
12.6.13	Number of adolescent/adult deaths due to known chronic disease	
12.6.14	Number of adolescent/adult deaths due to causes not known	
12.7	**Deaths due to Vector Borne Diseases (all age groups)**	
12.7.1	Number of deaths due to malaria-*Plasmodium vivax*	
12.7.2	Number of Deaths due to malaria-*Plasmodium falciparum*	

HMIS IN INDIA

Records and Registers

At present, the national health programmes have their independent HMIS; however, at the level of village and subcentre, the reports are generated by subcentre health team. The key registers at subcentre level are:

  A. Survey registers
   1. Subcentre village information
   2. Household information
   3. Eligible couple and children information

  B. Continuous care registers
   1. Family welfare services—tracking of eligible couples
   2. Maternal care services—tracking of pregnant women
   3. Child care and immunization services—tracking of children

 4. Tuberculosis and leprosy control

 5. Malaria and blood smear and treatment

C. Other registers

 1. Home visit diary

 2. Clinic register (common ailments)

 3. Stock and issue register

 4. Birth and death register

 5. Accounts of untied funds and JSY *(Janani Suraksha Yojna)*

Attempts have been made by several states to reduce the number of registers and records. Now integrated RCH register has been introduced. Similarly, Anganwadi workers have eleven set of registers like household survey register, birth and death register, beneficiary register for mother and children, immunization, growth charts and weight book and stock registers. ASHAs are also maintaining survey and service registers separately.

Reports

The subcentre ANMs, Anganwadi workers and ASHAs are the responsibility centres for HMIS and they prepare monthly reports. The subcentre report provides information on inputs (health workers, material equipment, monthly stock position of drugs, vaccines received, functional status of equipment, etc.). It also provides information on processes and outputs or performance in terms of antenatal care, natal care, pregnancy outcome, postnatal care, newborn care, referral services, STI/RTI detection, immunization, disease surveillance, contraception services, malaria and tuberculosis output, and data on impact indicators like births and deaths. It also has information on interaction with the community, besides general information on population and eligible couples—parity-wise and age-wise. Similarly, Anganwadi worker provides useful information on health and nutrition services and impact measurement.

This information is generated every month and sent to PHC. The feedback on this information is provided at the sector level (circle) monthly meeting of health workers, Anganwadi workers (AWWs) ASHAs and their supervisors.

Similarly, subcentre action plans are evolved at the level of subcentre once a year and submitted to higher levels. Monthly single updated reporting format for sub centre and equivalent institutions has been evolved to provide regular data/information to guide actions and decision making.

10

Medical Genetics

Out of every 100 babies born in India annually 6–7 have birth defects. Rashtriya Bal Swasthya Karyakram (RBSK) has been launched in India for screening and early interventions services under NHM in 2013. This new initiative aims at screening 0–18 years children for defects at birth, disease, deficiency and development delays for follow up and early intervention at district early intervention centre.

National Level Data of RBSK—2016-17 for Top Ten Diseases/ Detects

1. Dental problems 40.7%
2. Skin problems 25.17%
3. Visual impairment 11.26%
4. Severe anaemia 11%
5. Reactive air way disease 10.91%
6. Middle ear infection 8.18%
7. Vit A deficiency 3.79%
8. Language delay 1.27%
9. Convulsive disorders 1.17%
10. Congenital heart disease 1.03%

11

Medical Entomology and Control of Vectors of Diseases

Integrated control of vectors of diseases is an ideal control measure to control the population of vectors of diseases. The most practical and sustained measure to control vectors of diseases is **Environmental Control**, i.e. environment modification and environment manipulation by effective community participation with the aim of source reduction preventing breeding of vector or insects at household and community level; besides town planning and better housing. "Swachh Bharat Abhiyan" programme is a thrust area for control of vectors of diseases.

Source reduction, i.e. elimination of breeding of vectors

1. By environmental manipulation (temporary methods) minor engineering methods, deweeding, desilting, leveling, household waste water management by kitchen garden and soak pits, draining of water from coolers, draining of pots, covering overhead tanks, observing dry days, etc. can be effective measures to prevent vector breeding by **people themselves**.

2. **By environmental modification:** This means habitat modification. These are measures of permanent alteration of environments and long lasting such as physical transformation of land, water and vegetation, surface water drainage, filling and land reclamation and solid waste management by municipal authorities.

12
Epidemiology of Communicable Diseases and Related National Health Programmes

LINKED CONFIDENTIAL TESTING IN HIV SENTINEL SURVEILLANCE SYSTEM 2017

In antenatals and high risk groups until now unlinked annonymous strategy for HIV sentinel surveillance was being followed in the country. From 2017 onwards linked confidential testing system has been adopted in the country.

FOR ANTENATAL CLINIC SITES

Every pregnant women in India is expected to receive services as per the essential antenatal care package. The package includes minimum of at least four ANCs including early registration and first ANC in first trimester along with physical and abdominal examinations, Hb estimation and urine investigation, 2 doses of TT, consumption of IFA tablets (6 months during ANC and 6 months during PNC) and **universal screening/testing of pregnant women for HIV and syphilis** to eliminate transmission of syphilis and HIV (parent to child transmission).

- A portion of blood specimen collected for routine clinical diagnosis is separated for HIV surveillance purpose after removing all personal identifiers. The surveillance portion of the **specimen is coded.** No personal identifiers like name, address and mobile number is put on the vial containing HSS aliquot.
- The surveillance code is linked with ANC registration/OPD code in a separate register (HSS register) which is kept confidentially at the ANC HSS site.
- In high risk groups (HRG) the surveillance code is linked with TI unique ID code in a separate confidential register (HSS register) at HRG site.
- Report of the routine diagnostic tests (Hb-syphilis-blood group, urine/HIV) is communicated to the participants.

- The surveillance specimen is sent to the HSS testing or HSS DBS testing lab. Results of surveillance specimen reactive either for HIV or syphilis are shared with SACS ICTC in charge at the earliest. SACS/ICTC incharge coordinates with respective ANC site-incharge to refer cases for PPTCT services which were reactive in surveillance but not tested under the programme. This will facilitate offering of counselling, testing and or treatment services to pregnant women in order to keep them healthy and to protect their unborn baby. Similar approach is adopted for high risk groups.

ELIMINATION OF PARENT TO CHILD TRANSMISSION (EPTCT) OF SYPHILIS AND HIV IN INDIA BY 2020

There are many adverse outcomes due to maternal syphilis—like spontaneous abortions, stillbirth, low birth weight, congenital syphilis and even neonatal mortality. Congenital syphilis is a serious but preventable disease, which can be eliminated proactively through effective **screening of all pregnant women for syphilis** and treatment of those infected, including their partner and newborn. The syphilis sero-prevalence in India is 0.38%.

Key Strategies

  i. Ensuring universal ANC check up in more than 95% of antenatals.
 ii. Testing of syphilis and HIV together and both the tests to be essential tests in ANC service package.
iii. Treatment of all sero-reactive mothers, partners and newborn for syphilis.
 iv. Reporting and line listing of all cases of maternal syphilis and HIV and institutional delivery for them. Follow up of newborn up to 18 months of age.
  v. Making available supply of syphilis test kits and HIV test kits and Inj. benzathine penicillin, etc.
 vi. Scaling up testing—"Point of care test" with newer and simple technologies.

National Strategy of Prevention of Parent to Child Transmission (PPTCT) of HIV

Objective

Universal HIV testing every pregnant women in the country to "Eliminate parent to child transmission of HIV" and "elimination of new HIV infections among children by 2020.

National Aids Control Organization has implemented updated guidelines of life long ART (triple drug regimen) for all pregnant and lactating women living with HIV, regardless of CD4 count or

WHO clinical stage or duration of pregnancy, both for their own health and to prevent vertical HIV transmission. Babies born to HIV positive mothers are given Nevirapine single dose daily for 6 weeks and the exposed babies are followed up to 18 months for early infant diagnosis.

NATIONAL STRATEGIC PLAN AND "MISSION SAMPARK" 2017–24 (SUSTAINABLE DEVELOPMENT GOALS FOR HIV/AIDS BY 2030

Sustainable Development Goal for HIV/AIDS—Phase V of NACP "End the HIV/AIDS epidemic by 2030".

Definition: End the AIDS epidemic by 2030 is defined as 90% reduction of new HIV infections and AIDS related mortality, compared to base year of 2010.

Fast Track Targets by 2020 in NACP-India
- 90 – 90 – 90 treatment target by 2020.
  - i. 90% of all people living with HIV will know their HIV status.
  - ii. 90% of all people with diagnosed HIV infection will receive sustained antiretroviral therapy.
  - iii. 90 of all people receiving antiretroviral therapy will have durable viral suppression to the extent that it cannot replicate.

Incidence
- 75% reduction in new infections by 2020 from the current levels (base year 2010).
- Elimination of parent to child transmission of HIV and syphilis and new infections in children by universal coverage of pregnant mothers.

Zero-discrimination
By 2020 less than 10% of people living with or affected by HIV are discriminated within community and less than 10% of general population report discriminatory attitudes towards people living with HIV. Recently passed HIV/AIDS prevention and control bill 2017, paves the way for right to education, livelihood and residence to PLHIV.

India Scorecard
- Out of 21.2 lakh PL HIV about 14.2 lakh (67%) are aware of their HIV status.
- Out of 21 lakh persons living with HIV (PLHIV) 11.5 Lakh (55%) were on ART.

- Data on the number of PL HIV on ART who are virally suppressed is not available because of lack of viral load testing labs.
- From 2007 to 2015 there has been 33% reduction in new HIV infections.
- The programme has reached to 42% of pregnant women in the country. Utilization of ANC in Government sector is low.
- National IBBS conducted in 2015 among key populations showed that 27% of FSW, 17% MSM and 46% IDU reported discrimination by family, friends and neighbours.

NATIONAL STRATEGIC PLAN AND MISSION "SAMPARK" 2017–24

Speed up detection of hidden HIV positive cases, ensure high coverage of targeted population by improved linkage with STI, TB and TI. Reframe targeted interventions to trace those left to followup:
- Roll out newer initiatives such as community based testing for key populations to track hidden HIV positives and help fast track treatment.
- Population prioritization and geoprioritization for high yield.
- Integration with NHM/RCH and ICDS to reach out to pregnant women to scale up PPTCT for elimination of parent to child transmission of HIV and syphilis.
- Adoption of WHO guidelines to introduce "Test and Treat" for key populations and sero-discordant couples.
- Strengthening of infrastrcuture, human resources and laboratory component as also logistics.

SYNDROMIC CASE MANAGEMENT—NATIONAL GUIDELINES ON RTI/STI

Definition

A syndrome is defined as a group of consistent common symptoms and signs caused by more than one organism. An STI/RTI syndrome is a combination of symptoms and signs typically associated with sexually transmitted microorganisms, e.g. **genital ulcer disease syndrome,** which may be due to syphilis, chancroid, herpes simplex, etc.

Aim

The aim of STI/RTI syndromic case management is to identify the syndrome correctly and manage them accordingly. Syndromic diagnosis leads to immediate treatment for all of the most important possible causative agents. This is important because mixed infections occur frequently in STI/RTI. Besides, syndromic management of STI/RTI can effectively treat cases in settings with limited or no **laboratory facilities**. This means syndromic treatment can quickly render the patient non-infectious.

Overview of STI/RTI

Sexually transmitted infections (STI) and reproductive tract infections (RTI) have a major impact on sexual and reproductive health. As per the World Health Organization (WHO), globally 499 million new episodes of **curable sexually transmitted infections** (syphilis, gonorrhoea, chlamydia and trichomoniasis) occur yearly (2008 estimates); a significant proportion of these infections are occurring in developing countries. Sexually transmitted infections are an important **cause of infertility in men and women**. In pregnant women with untreated early syphilis, **21% of pregnancies result** in stillbirth and **9% in neonatal deaths.** Drug resistance, especially for gonorrhoea, is a major threat to STI control globally. Some STI can increase the risk of HIV acquisition and transmission by **three-fold or more.**

Of the more than 30 identified pathogens known to be transmitted sexually, syphilis, gonorrhoea, chlamydia, trichomoniasis, human immunodeficiency virus (HIV), Human papilloma virus (HPV), herpes simplex virus (HSV), and hepatitis B virus (HBV) have been linked to the greatest incidence of illness.

Sexually transmitted infections/Reproductive tract infections (STI/RTI) are an important public health problem in India. A community based STI/RTI prevalence study conducted during 2002–03 by the Indian Council of Medical Research (ICMR) has shown that 6% of the adult population in India has one or more STI/RTI. This amounts to occurrence of about 30–35 million episodes of STI/RTI every year in the country. Controlling STI/RTI helps to decrease HIV infection rates and provides a window of opportunity for counselling on HIV prevention and improving sexual and reproductive health.

Currently, the available data from the STI/RTI control and prevention programme suggests a significant decline of bacterial STIs (syphilis, gonorrhoea). Chancroid is almost on the verge of disappearance. On the other hand, viral STIs (herpes, genital warts, hepatitis B) are showing an increasing trend. There is a significant burden of lower RTI (trichomoniasis, bacterial vaginosis and candidiasis) among women with no evidence to suggest a decline in their prevalence, thus affecting the quality of their reproductive health.

Essential Steps of STI/RTI Syndromic Case Management
(*See* Flowcharts 12.1–12.4)

The essential steps of STI/RTI syndromic case management include:
1. **History:** Chief complaints or symptoms—Assess risks by: History of recent unprotected sex and sex of partner:
   - Multiple sexual partners.
   - Recent change in sexual partners.

- Partner with symptoms suggestive of STI in recent past.
- Type of exposure-oral, vaginal and anal.
2. Clinical examination: Genital/oral and ano-rectal apart from general examination.
3. Appropriate syndromic diagnosis as per syndromic flowcharts.
4. Minimal laboratory tests, wherever available.
5. Early and effective treatment, preferably single dose and directly observed treatment (DOT).
6. Promotion and provision of condoms.
7. Counselling for behaviour change and risk reduction.
8. Referral for syphilis screening and voluntary HIV counselling and testing.
9. Partner/s notification and management.
10. Follow-up as per schedule.
11. Documentation of case details and laboratory results.

FROM "STOP TB" STRATEGY TO "END TB" STRATEGY BY 2030

From 2017 onward the Goal is to "End Global TB Epidemic" by implementing "the end TB strategy". Adopted by the World Health Assembly in may 2014 with targets linked to the newly adopted "Sustainable Development Goals" the strategy serves as a blue print for countries to Achieve followings from base year 2015.

- Reduce TB deaths by 90% by 2030.
- Reduce TB incidence by 80% and
- Reduce TB prevalence by 80%
- Achieve treatment success rate in DSTB 92%.
- Achieve treatment success rate in DRTB 95%
- Ensure elimination of catastrophic costs due to TB by 2030, compared with 2015.
- In line with the above objectives National strategic Plan (NSP) from 2017 to 2025 has been evolved for elimination of TB.

Burden of TB Disease in India 2015

Tuberculosis is a global problem and distributed worldwide. India is high burden country for TB along with Indonesia China, Nigeria Pakistan and South Africa. Out of 10.4 million new cases worldwide in 2015 India contributed 2.8 million cases (27% of global incidence) (Fig. 12.1 and Table 12.1) WHO in 1993 declared TB as global emergency.

Flowcharts for Management of RTI/STI Syndromes

Flowchart 12.1: Management of urethral discharge/burning micturition in males

SYNDROME: URETHRAL DISCHARGE IN MALES

RTIs/STIs: GONORRHOEA, CHLAMYDIAL INFECTION, TRICHOMONIASIS

Causative organisms
- *Neisseria gonorrhoeae*
- *Chlamydia trachomatis*
- *Trichomonas vaginalis*
- Other organisms

History of
- Urethral discharge
- Pain or burning while passing urine, increased frequency of urination
- Sexual exposure of either partner to high-risk practices like orogenital sex in previous 2 months
- Assess risk behaviours

Examination—Look for
- The urethral meatus for redness and swelling
- Presence of urethral discharge
- If urethral discharge is not seen, then gently massage the urethra from the ventral part of the penis towards the meatus and look for thick, creamy greenish-yellow or mucoid discharge

Laboratory investigations (if available)
- Gram stain examination of the urethral smear will show gram-negative intracellular diplococci in case of gonorrhea
- In case of non-gonococcal urethritis more than 5 neutrophils per oil immersion field (1000X) in the urethral smear or more than 10 neutrophils per high power field in the sediment of the first void urine
- RPR test for syphilis

Treatment—Colour coded Kit 1 Grey

As dual infection is common, the treatment for urethral discharge should adequately cover therapy for both gonorrhoea and chlamydial infections

Recommended regimen for uncomplicated urethral discharge (UD) syndrome

Uncomplicated infections indicate that the disease is limited to the anogenital region (anterior urethritis and proctitis)

- Tab. cefixime 400 mg orally, single dose **plus**
- Tab. azithromycin 1 g orally single dose under supervision or
  Cap doxycycline 100 mg twice a day for 7 days
- Advise the client to return after 7 days of start of therapy
- Patients who have UD syndrome and also are infected with HIV should receive the same treatment regimen as those who are HIV negative

(Contd...)

When symptoms persist (discharge or only dysuria persists after 7 days) after adequate treatment for gonorrhoea and chlamydia in the index client and partner(s), they should be treated for *Trichomonas vaginalis*

- Tab. Secnidazole 2 g orally, single dose (to treat for *T. vaginalis*)

If the symptoms still persists

- Refer to higher centre as early as possible

If individuals are allergic to azithromycin, give erythromycin 500 mg four times a day for 7 days

Syndrome specific guidelines for partner management

Treat all sexual partners of patients in past 2 months

- Treat female partners on same lines after ruling out pregnancy and history of allergies
- Advise sexual abstinence during the course of treatment
- Provide condoms, educate about correct and consistent use
- Refer for voluntary counselling and testing for HIV, syphilis and hepatitis B

Follow-up: After seven days

- To see reports of tests done for HIV, syphilis
- If symptoms/signs persist assess whether it is due to trichomonas infection, if possible treat with tab secnidazole 2 gm orally
- If symptoms and signs persist, assess whether it is due to treatment failure or re-infection and advise prompt referral if required

Management of pregnant partner

Pregnant partners of male clients with urethral discharge should be examined by doing a per speculum as well as a per vaginal examination and should be treated with:

- Cephalosporins to cover gonococcal infection are safe and effective in pregnancy
- Tab. cefixime 400 mg orally, single dose **OR** ceftriaxone 250 mg by intramuscular injection **PLUS**

Tab. Azithromycin 1 gm stat orally **OR**

- Tab. erythromycin 500 mg orally four times a day for 7 days **OR**

Cap. amoxycillin 500 mg orally, three times a day for 7 days to cover chlamydial infection

Note: Quinolones (like ofloxacin, ciprofloxacin), doxycycline are contraindicated in pregnant women

Recurrent and persistent urethritis-recommended treatment: Objective signs of urethritis should be present before start of trt

- Metronidazole 2 gm orally in a single dose **OR**
- Tinidazole 2 gm orally in a single dose **PLUS**
- Azithromycin 1 gm orally in a single dose (if not used for initial episode)

Flowchart 12.2: Management of genital ulcer disease (non herpetic and herpetic syndrome)

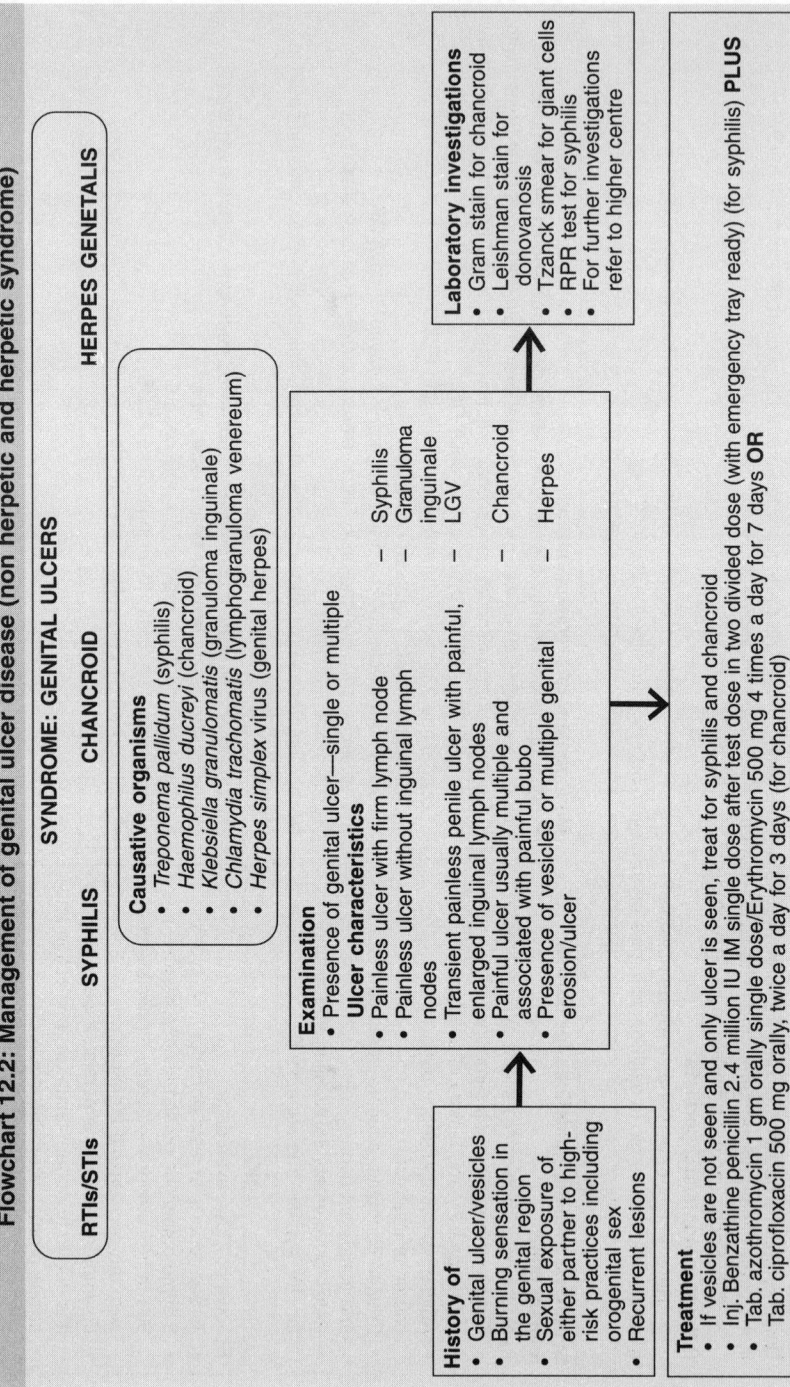

RTIs/STIs

SYNDROME: GENITAL ULCERS

SYPHILIS   **CHANCROID**   **HERPES GENETALIS**

Causative organisms
- *Treponema pallidum* (syphilis)
- *Haemophilus ducreyi* (chancroid)
- *Klebsiella granulomatis* (granuloma inguinale)
- *Chlamydia trachomatis* (lymphogranuloma venereum)
- *Herpes simplex virus* (genital herpes)

Examination
- Presence of genital ulcer—single or multiple

Ulcer characteristics
- Painless ulcer with firm lymph node — Syphilis
- Painless ulcer without inguinal lymph — Granuloma
  nodes   inguinale
- Transient painless penile ulcer with painful, — LGV
  enlarged inguinal lymph nodes
- Painful ulcer usually multiple and — Chancroid
  associated with painful bubo
- Presence of vesicles or multiple genital — Herpes
  erosion/ulcer

Laboratory investigations
- Gram stain for chancroid
- Leishman stain for
  donovanosis
- Tzanck smear for giant cells
- RPR test for syphilis
- For further investigations
  refer to higher centre

History of
- Genital ulcer/vesicles
- Burning sensation in
  the genital region
- Sexual exposure of
  either partner to high-
  risk practices including
  orogenital sex
- Recurrent lesions

Treatment
- If vesicles are not seen and only ulcer is seen, treat for syphilis and chancroid
- Inj. Benzathine penicillin 2.4 million IU IM single dose after test dose in two divided dose (with emergency tray ready) (for syphilis) **PLUS**
- Tab. azothromycin 1 gm orally single dose/Erythromycin 500 mg 4 times a day for 7 days **OR**
  Tab. ciprofloxacin 500 mg orally, twice a day for 3 days (for chancroid)

(Contd...)

- In individuals allergic to or intolerant to penicillin
  - Cap doxycycline 100 mg orally, twice daily for 15 days **OR**
  - Tab. azithromycin 2 gm as a single dose to treat early syphilis
- If vescicles or multiple painful ulcers are present treat for herpes
- In primary episode and for recurrence-Tab. Acyclovir 400 mg TDS for 7 days.

Syndrome specific guidelines for partner management

- Partners should be treated for syphilis and chancroid with same regimen
- Treat all partners who are in contact with client in last 3 months prior to the onset of ulcer
- No partner treatment for herpes (in the absence of active episode/lesions)
- Advise sexual abstinence during the course of treatment
- Provide condoms, educate about correct and consistent use
- Refer for voluntary counselling and testing for HIV, syphilis and hepatitis B
- Schedule return visit after 7 days

Kit 3: White: Genital ulcer, non-herpetic ulcers

Kit 4: Blue: Patient allergic to penicillin, non-herpetic ulcer

Kit 5: Red: Herpetic ulcers

Management of pregnant women

- Quinolones (like ofloxacin, ciprofloxacin), doxycycline, sulfonamides are contraindicated in pregnant women
- Pregnant women who test positive for RPR in any dilution should be considered infected and should be provided treatment for syphilis unless adequate treatment is documented in the medical records and sequential serologic antibody titers have declined
- Inj Benzathine penicillin 2.4 million IU IM after test dose (with emergency tray ready)
- Pregnant women who are allergic to penicillin should be treated with erythromycin and the neonate should be treated for syphilis after delivery
- Tab. erythromycin 500 mg orally four times a day for 15 days
  (Note: Erythromycin estolate is contraindicated in pregnancy because of drug related hepatotoxicity. Only erythromycin base or erythromycin ethyl succinate should be used in pregnancy)
- All pregnant women should be asked history of genital herpes and examined carefully for herpetic lesions
- Women without symptoms or signs of genital herpes or its prodrome can deliver vaginally
- Women with genital herpetic lesions at the onset of labour should be delivered by caesarean section to prevent neonatal herpes
- Acyclovir may be administered orally to pregnant women with first episode genital herpes or severe recurrent herpes
- Pregnant women should be given Tab Acyclovir 400 mg TDs during last 4 weeks of pregnancy

Flowchart 12.3: Management of vaginal and cervical discharge syndrome

SYNDROME: VAGINAL DISCHARGE

| VAGINITIS | CERVICITIS | CERVICAL HERPES | TRICHOMONIASIS |

Causative organisms
Vaginitis
- *Trichomonas vaginalis* (TV)
- *Candida albicans*
- Multiple organisms *Gardnerella vaginalis, Mycoplasma,* ureaplasma and anaerobes

Causative organisms
Cervicitis
- *Trichomonas vaginalis*
- *Neisseria gonorrhoeae*
- *Chlamydia trachomatis*
- *Herpes simplex virus*
- Human papilloma virus

History
- Menstrual history to rule out pregnancy
- Nature and type of discharge (amount, smell, color, consistency)
- Genital itching
- Burning while passing urine, increased frequency
- Presence of any ulcer, swelling on the vulval or inguinal region
- Genital complaints in sexual partners
- Low backache
- Assess risk

Examination
- Per speculum followed by bimanual examination to differentiate between vaginitis and cervicitis and to rule out PID
  (a) *Vaginitis:* The clasic clinical presentations
    - Trichomoniasis—greenish frothy discharge
    - Candidiasis—curdy white discharge
    - Bacterial vaginosis—adherent discharge
    - Mixed infections may present with atypical discharge
  (b) *Cervicitis signs:* Frequently asymptomatic
- Erythematous cervix
- Mucopurulent cervical discharge
- If speculum examination is not possible or client is hesitant treat both for vaginitis and cervicitis

Laboratory investigations
(if available)
- Wet mount microscopy of the discharge for *Trichomonas vaginalis*
- 10% KOH preparation for *Candida albicans*
- Gram stain of vaginal smear clue cells seen in bacterial vaginosis
- Gram stain of endocervical smear to detect gonococci
- RPR test for syphilis
- Refer to ICTC for counselling and testing
- Microscopic examination of vaginal fluid for WBC > 10

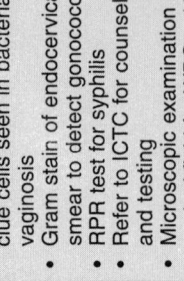
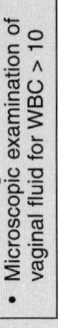

(Contd...)

Kit 2: Green

Treatment

Vaginitis (TV + BV + Candida)

- Tab. secnidazole 2 g orally, single dose **or**
  Tab. tinidazole 500 mg orally, twice daily for 5 days **or** Tablet metronidazol 400 mg twice daily for 7 days
- Treat for candidiasis with Tab. fluconazole 150 mg orally single dose **or** local clotrimazole 500 mg vaginal pessary once
- Pregnancy, diabetes, HIV may also be influencing factors and should be considered in recurrent infections

Treatment for cervical infection (chlamydia and gonorrhoea)

- Tab. cefixime 400 mg orally, single dose **Plus**
  Azithromycin 1 gram, 1 hour before food. If vomiting within 1 hour, give anti-emetic and repeat treatment
  - If vaginitis and cervicitis are present together treat for both
  - Instruct client to avoid douching and avoid alcohol consumption during metronidazole therapy
  - Follow-up after one week to document symptomatic cure and results of HIV/syphilis tests

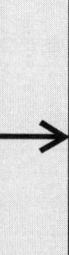

Management in pregnant women

Per speculum examination should be done to rule out pregnancy, complications like abortion, premature rupture of membranes

Treatment for vaginitis (TV + BV + Candida)

In first trimester of pregnancy

- Local treatment with clotrimazole vaginal pessary/cream only for candidiasis. Oral fluconazole is contraindicated in pregnancy
- Tablet metronidazole 400 mg bid for 7 days for BV or TV

Management of preganant women for cervicitis: Same as in non preganant women

Follow up after 7 days: To document symptomatic cure and results of HIV and syphilis tests

Specific guidelines for partner management

For vaginitis due to BV and Candida:

- Not required
- Treat current partner only if no improvement after initial treatment
- If partner is symptomatic, treat client and partner using above protocols

For cervicitis and trichomonas infection:

- Treat all sexual partners in the last 30 days with above protocols
- Advise sexual abstinence during the course of treatment
- Schedule return visit after 7 days

Flowchart 12.4: Management of lower abdominal pain (LAP) syndrome in females

LAP syndrome comprises a spectrum of inflammatory disorders of the upper female genital tract, including any combination of endometritis, salpingitis, tubo-ovarian abscess and pelvic peritonitis.

Pelvic inflammatory disease (PID)

Causative organisms
- *Neisseria gonorrhoeae*
- *Chlamydia trachomatis*
- *Mycoplasma*, *Gardnerella*, Anaerobic bacteria (*Bacteroides* sp, gram-positive cocci)

History of
- Lower abdominal pain
- Fever
- Vaginal discharge
- Menstrual irregularities like heavy, irregular vaginal bleeding
- Dysmenorrhoea
- Dyspareunia
- Dysuria, tenesmus
- Low backache
- Contraceptive use like IUD
- Assess risks

Examination
- General examination: Temperature, pulse, blood pressure
- Per speculum examination: Vaginal/cervical discharge, congestion or ulcers
- Per abdominal examination: Lower abdominal tenderness or guarding
- Pelvic examination: Uterine/adnexal tenderness, cervical movement, tenderness

Note: A urine pregnancy test should be done in all women suspected of having PID to rule out ectopic pregnancy

Laboratory investigations if available
- Wet smear examination
- Gram stain for gonorrhoea
- Complete blood count and ESR
- Urine microscopy for pus
- RPR test for syphilis
- Refer to ICTC

Differential diagnosis
- Ectopic pregnancy
- Twisted ovarian cyst
- Ovarian tumor
- Appendicitis
- Abdominal tuberculosis

(Contd...)

Treatment (outpatient treatment)　　　　　　　**Kit 6:** Yellow

In mild or moderate PID (in the absence of tubo-ovarian abscess), out patient treatment can be given

Therapy is required to cover *Neisseria gonorrhoeae*, *Chlamydia trachomatis* and anaerobes

- Tab. cefixime 400 mg orally STAT **PLUS**
- Tab. metronidazole 400 mg orally, twice daily for 14 days (to treat anaerobic infection) **PLUS**
- Doxycycline, 100 mg orally, twice a day for 2 weeks (to treat chlamydial infection)
- Tab. ibuprofen 400 mg orally, three times a day for 3–5 days
- Tab. ranitidine 150 mg orally, twice daily to prevent gastritis
- Remove intrauterine device, if present, under antibiotic cover of 24–48 hours
- Advise abstinence during the course of treatment and educate on correct and consistent use of condoms
- Observe for 3 days. If no improvement (i.e. absence of fever, reduction in abdominal tenderness, reduction in cervical movement, adnexal and uterine tenderness) or if symptoms worsen, refer for inpatient treatment

Avoid alcohol consumption during metronidazole therapy

Caution: PID can be a serious condition. Refer the client to the hospital if she does not respond to treatment within 3 days and even earlier if her condition worsens

Syndrome specific guidelines for partner management

- Treat all male sexual partners in past 2 months
- Treat male partners for urethral discharge (gonorrhoea and chlamydia)
- Advise sexual abstinence during the course of treatment
- Provide condoms, educate on correct and consistent use
- Refer for voluntary counselling and testing for HIV, syphilis and hepatitis B
- Inform about the complications if left untreated and sequelae
- Schedule return visit after 3 days, 7 days and 14 days to ensure compliance, document sympatomatic cure and results of HIV and syphilis tests

Management of pregnant women

Though PID is rare in pregnancy

➢ Any pregnant woman suspected to have PID should be referred to district hospital for hospitalization and treated with a parenteral regimen which would be safe in pregnancy

➢ Doxycycline is contraindicated in pregnancy

Key counselling messages:

- Educate and counsel client and sexual partners on STI/RTI and complete treatment
- Treat partners as per syndrome
- Provide condoms and their correct and consistent use

Hospitalization of clients with acute PID should be seriously considered when:

- The diagnosis is uncertain
- Surgical emergencies, e.g. appendicitis or ectopic pregnancy cannot be excluded
- A pelvic abscess is suspected
- Severe illness precludes management on an outpatient basis
- The woman is pregnant
- The client is unable to follow or tolerate an outpatient regimen
- The client has failed to respond to outpatient therapy

Note: All clients requiring hospitalization should be referred to the district hospital

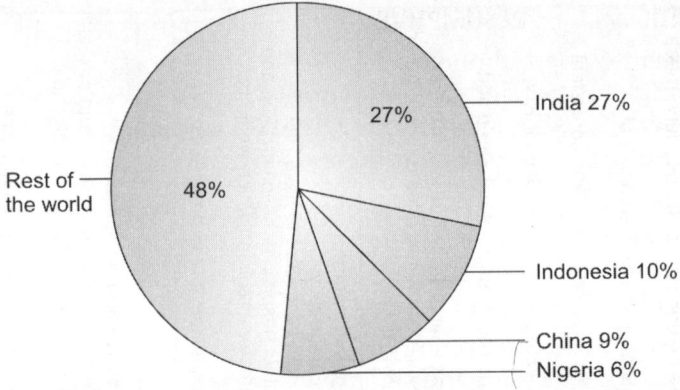

Fig. 12.1: India's share in global incidence of TB 2015

Table 12.1: TB disease burden in India and trends of TB			
		Period	
Indicators	*1958–60*	*2000*	*2014–2015*
Total population in million	430	1000	1311
Burden of TB in million	9	8.5	2.5
Bacillary cases (pulmonary TB) in million	3.60	3.80	1.2

Incidence

India has highest burden of both TB and MDR TB and second highest of HIV associated TB. An estimated 2.8 million New cases of TB and 130000 cases of MDR-TB emerge annually in India. Disease burden in 2014 was estimated at 2.5 million (Prevalence) cases; out of which 1.2 million were bacillary cases[1-4]. National level surveys done in 1958 and year 2000 indicated high burden (Prevalence) of 8.5 to 9 million cases and the case load has declined over the years to about 2.5 million cases[5], because of programme interventions. To estimate exact prevalence (Disease burden).

INDIA IS CONDUCTING ITS FIRST NATIONAL TUBERCULOSIS PREVALENCE SURVEY IN 2018

CASE FINDING AND DIAGNOSIS STRATEGY

To achieve universal access to early accurate diagnosis of TB and enhancing case finding efficiency, **identification of presumptive TB cases** at the first **point of care** and linking them to the best available diagnostic tests is of paramount importance. Early case detection is vital to interrupt the transmission of TB disease.

DEFINITIONS OF PRESUMPTIVE TB

1. Presumptive pulmonary TB refers to a person with any of the symptoms and signs suggestive of TB including **cough >2 weeks, fever >2 weeks, significant weight loss, haemoptysis,** and **any abnormality in chest radiograph.**

   Note: In addition, contacts of microbiologically confirmed TB patients, PLHIV, diabetics, malnourished, cancer patients, patients on immune-suppressants or steroids should be regularly **screened** for signs and symptoms of TB.

2. Presumptive extra pulmonary TB refers to the presence of organ specific symptoms and signs like swelling of lymph node, pain and swelling in joints, neck stiffness, disorientation, etc. and/or constitutional symptoms like significant weight loss, persistent fever for 2 weeks, and night sweats.[3]

3. Presumptive paediatric TB refers to children with persistent fever and/or cough for more than 2 weeks, loss of weight*/no weight gain and/or history of contact with infectious TB cases**.

4. Presumptive DR TB refers to those TB patients who have failed treatment with first line drugs, paediatric TB non responders, TB patients who are contacts of DR-TB (or Rif resistance), TB patients who are found positive on any follow-up sputum smear examination during treatment with first line drugs, previously treated TB cases, and TB patients with HIV co-infection.

DIAGNOSTIC TOOLS

Tools for microbiological confirmation of TB.

All efforts should be undertaken for microbiologically confirming the diagnosis in presumptive TB patients. Under RNTCP, the acceptable methods for microbiological diagnosis of TB are:

1. Sputum smear microscopy (for AFB)
   - Ziehl-Neelsen staining
   - Fluorescence staining

---

* History of unexplained weight loss or no weight gain in past 3 months; loss of weight is defined as loss of more than 5% body weight as compared to highest weight recorded in last 3 months.

** In a symptomatic child, contact with a person with any form of active TB within last 2 years may be significant.

2. Sputum culture—it is highly sensitive and specific (Gold Standard), but requires 2–8 weeks to yield results and hence alone does not help in early diagnosis.

3. Cartridge based nucleic acid amplification test (CBNAAT) provides accurate and rapid diagnosis of TB by detecting *Mycobacterium tuberculosis* and rifampicin resistance within one hour.

4. Chest X-ray (CXR)—it is used as a screening tool to increase the sensitivity of diagnostic algorithm.

Diagnostic Algorithm for Pulmonary TB[17] (Fig. 12.2)

a. All presumptive TB (specifically for PTB symptoms) will undergo sputum smear examination (ZN/LEDFM). Two specimens will be collected (spot-early morning or spot-spot). If the first smear is positive and the patient is not at risk for Drug Resistant (DR) TB, he will be categorized as microbiologically confirmed TB (sensitivity status not known).

b. Smear positive and presumptive MDR TB (as per PMDT guidelines) and in settings of high MDR TB (e.g. MDR TB rates >5% among new cases and >20% among re-treatment cases), a CBNAAT will be performed to rule out rifampicin resistance before initiation of treatment where patients will be categorized as microbiologically confirmed drug sensitive (DST) TB or RIF resistant TB.

c. If the first smear is negative, CXR may be considered and if reported as suggestive of TB, the 2nd sample will be subjected to smear and CBNAAT simultaneously.

d. Based on CBNAAT results, patients will be categorized as microbiologically confirmed drug sensitive TB or Rif resistant TB, if negative move to differential diagnosis for other etiology or point f.

e. A RIF indeterminate result will get an additional CBNAAT to get a valid result and in case of indeterminate on second occasion, an additional specimen will be collected and sent to the nearest Intermediate Reference Laboratory (IRL) or Culture and Drug Susceptibility Testing (C and DST) centre for LPA or liquid culture and DST as appropriate.

f. Wherever the facilities are available, efforts should be made to obtain DST results of all drugs by collecting additional samples and sending to nearest C and DST (subject to laboratory capacity).

g. If both sputum smears and CXR are negative, and physician is still suspecting TB, he will refer patient to pulmonology expert/chest specialist.

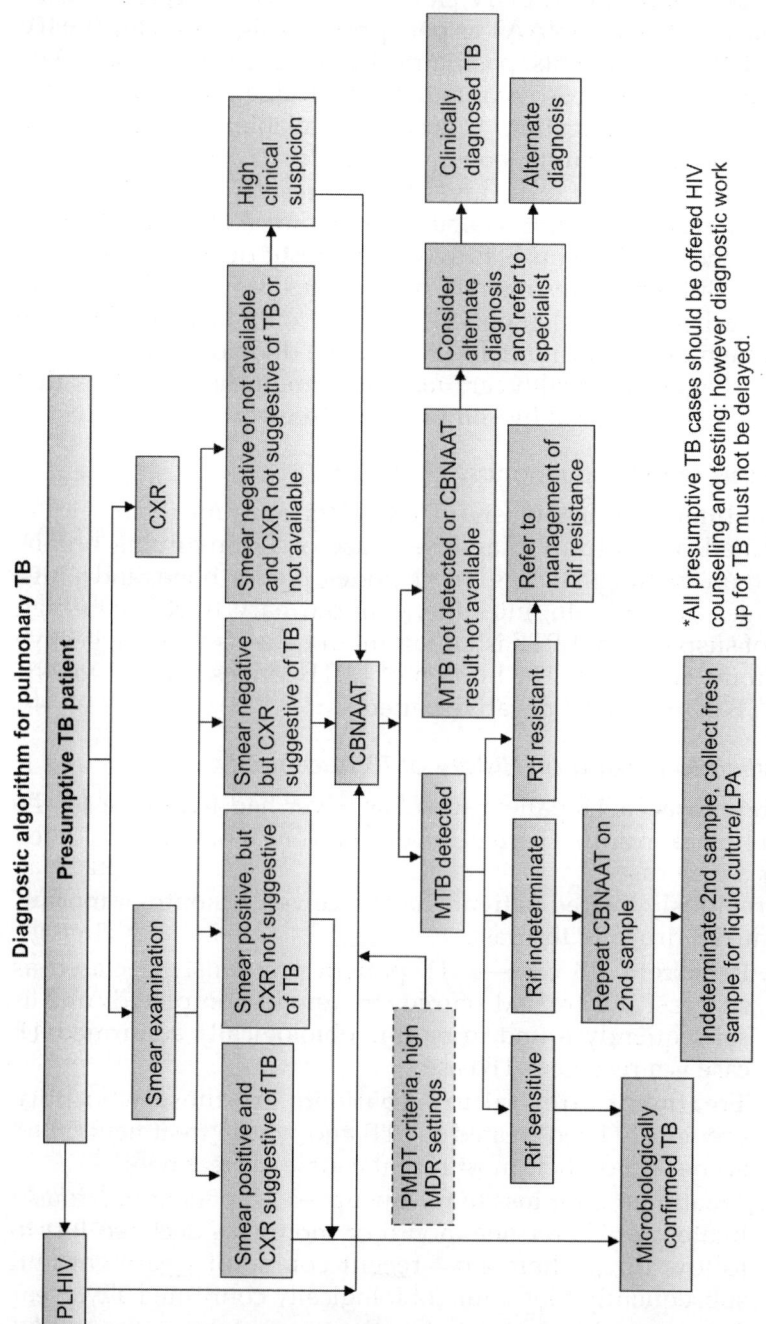

Fig. 12.2: Diagnostic algorithm for pulmonary TB

h. All key populations (PLHIV, children, EPTB, etc.) will preferentially get an upfront CBNAAT as per approved algorithm for PLHIV and TB HIV patients, paediatric TB and extra-pulmonary TB.

i. The algorithm does not mandatorily decide the "order to Do" the tests/investigation. If needed/available, appropriate test may be done simultaneously but "order of consideration" for different types of tests/investigation results should be as per the algorithm. (e.g. If available, smear for AFB and CXR may be done simultaneously to avoid diagnostic delay/patient's day loss. But, smear results will be prioritized over CXR to make an early diagnosis). If patient walks in with the latest CXR, the same may be considered to reduce the diagnostic delay.

j. All diagnositic health care facilities should have TB labs that are quality assured by competent authority.

Diagnosis of Extra-pulmonary TB (EPTB)

Extra pulmonary tuberculosis (EPTB) refers to any microbiologically confirmed or clinically diagnosed case of TB involving organs other than the lungs such as lymph nodes, pleura, bones and joints, meninges of the brain, intestine, genitourinary tract, etc. a high level of suspicion of EPTB is important in patients with suggestive symptoms and signs. The burden of EPTB ranges from 15 to 20% of all TB cases in HIV negative patients.

Classification Based on History of TB Treatment

a. **New case**—a TB patient who has never had treatment for TB or has taken anti-TB drugs for less than one month is considered as a new case.

b. **Previously treated patients** have received 1 month or more of anti-TB drugs in the past.

   i. **Recurrent TB case**—a TB patient previously declared as successfully treated (cured/treatment completed) and is subsequently found to be microbiologically confirmed TB case is a recurrent TB case.

   ii. **Treatment after failure**—patients are those who have previously been treated for TB and whose treatment failed at the end of their most recent course of treatment.

   iii. **Treatment after loss to follow up**—a TB patient previously treated for TB for one month or more was declared lost to follow up in their most recent course of treatment and subsequently found microbiologically confirmed TB case.

   iv. **Other previously treated patients** are those patients who have been previously treated for TB but whose outcome after their most recent course of treatment is unknown or undocumented.

c. **Transferred in:** A TB patient who is received for treatment in a Tuberculosis Unit, after registered for treatment in another TB unit is considered as a case of transferred in.

RNTCP Case Definitions

i. **Microbiologically confirmed TB case**—it refers to a presumptive TB patient with biological specimen positive for acid fast bacilli, or positive for *Mycobacterium tuberculosis* on culture, or positive for tuberculosis through Quality Assured Rapid Diagnostic Molecular test.

ii. **Clinically diagnosed TB case**—it refers to a presumptive TB patient who is not microbiologically confirmed, but has been diagnosed with active TB by a clinician on the basis of X-ray abnormalities, histopathology or clinical signs with a decision to treat the patient with a full course of anti-TB treatment.

Classification Based on Drug Resistance

a. **Mono-resistance (MR):** A TB patient, whose biological specimen is resistant to one first-line anti-TB drug only.

b. **Poly-drug resistance (PDR):** A TB patient, whose biological specimen is resistant to more than one first-line anti-TB drug, other than both INH and rifampicin.

c. **Multi drug resistance (MDR):** A TB patient, whose biological specimen is resistant to both isoniazid and rifampicin with or without resistance to other first line drugs, based on the results from a quality assured laboratory.

Rifampicin resistance (RR): Resistance to rifampicin detected using phenotypic or genotypic methods, with or without resistance to other anti-TB drugs excluding INH. Patients, who have any Rifampicin resistance, should also be managed as if they are MDR TB cases.

d. **Extensive drug resistance (XDR):** A MDR TB case whose biological specimen is additionally resistant to a fluoroquinolone (ofloxacin, levofloxacin, or moxifloxacin) and a second-line injectable anti TB drug (kanamycin, amikacin, or capreomycin) from a quality assured laboratory.

From Passive Case Detection to Passive Plus Active Case Detection

RNTCP has followed passive case detection strategy till 2016. Patient with cough with or without fever reported themselves to health facility (Govt or Private). This approach delays the diagnosis and treatment initiation. Active case finding approach significantly reduces the delay and initiation of treatment. **Active case finding** strategy has been implemented in 2017 across the country first in 50 high burden districts and later on extended to urban slums and rural areas to cover **vulnerable populations**. Programme also focuses on using rapid diagnostic tests to key vulnerable populations so that same day diagnosis and treatment can be initiated in paediatric, PL HIV and private notified patients.

Screening of High-Risk Populations and Areas—by Campaign

Contacts of microbiologically confirmed cases, people living with HIV (PLHIV), malnourished, diabetics, cancer patients, patients on immunosuppressant or maintenance steroid therapy, Silicosis and Kala-azar should regularly be screened for TB.

Enhanced case finding should be undertaken in **high-risk populations** such as healthcare workers, prisoners, slum dwellors, and miners, refugee camps, night shelters, old age homes, industrial workers, construction sites, difficult to reach villages and tribal areas, etc.

Activities in campaign include: mapping of high risk areas and vulnerable populations in urban and rural areas by health teams. House to house visits to cover most vulnerable to detect presumptive TB cases (suggestive symptoms and signs of TB) and collection of two sputum samples for microscopy at designated microscopic centre, followed by treatment.

DRUG REGIMEN FOR TREATMENT—DAILY REGIMEN

DRUG SENSITIVE TB

The RNTCP adopted thrice weekly regimen for treatment of drug sensitive TB until now. The programme is now introducing daily regimen for treatment of drug sensitive Tuberculosis among PLHIV and pediatric TB patients in the entire country and for all TB patients in 104 districts initially. The daily regimen now has been scaled up to the entire country in November 2017.

The principle of treatment for tuberculosis (other than confirmed Drug resistant forms of TB) with daily regimen is to administer daily fixed dose combinations of first—line anti-tuberculosis drugs in appropriate weight bands.

For new TB cases: The treatment in intensive phase (IP) will consist of 2 months of Isoniazid, Rifampicin, Pyrazinamide and Ethambutol in daily dosages as per four weight band categories.

There will be no need for extension of IP. Only Pyrazinamide will be stopped in the continuation phase (CP), while the other three drugs will be continued for another 4 months as daily dosages.

For previously treated cases of TB: The IP will be of 3 months, where injection Streptomycin will be stopped after 2 months and the remaining four drugs (INH, Rifampicin, Pyrazinamide and Ethambutol) in daily dosages as per weight bands will be continued for another one month. There will be no need for extension of IP. At the start of CP, Pyrazinamide will be stopped while the rest of the drugs—Rifampicin, INH and Ethambutol will be continued for another 5 months as daily dosages in the CP.

The CP in both new and previously treated cases may be extended by 3–6 months in certain forms of TB like CNS TB, Skeletal TB, Disseminated TB, etc. based on clinical decision of the treating physician. Extension beyond 12 weeks should only be on recommendation of experts of the concerned field. Loose Drugs would be needed as substitutions in case of adverse drug reaction or with co-morbid conditions.

Daily regimen for drug sensitive TB		
Type of TB case	Treatment regimen in IP	Treatment regimen CP
New	(2) HRZE	(4) HRE
Previously treated	(2) HRZES + (1) HRZE	(5) HRE

MDR/RR-TB Cases (Without Additional Resistance)

These patients are to be treated with standard treatment regimen for MDR-TB that contains 6 to 9 months of IP with Kanamycin, Levofloxacin, Ethambutol, Pyrazinamide, Ethionamide and Cycloserine and 18 months of CP with levofloxacin, Ethambutol, Ethionamide and Cycloserine.

MDR/RR-TB cases (without additional resistance)		
Type of TB case	Treatment regimen in IP	Treatment regimen CP
Rifampicin resistant + isoniazid sensitive or unknown	(6–9) Km LfxEto Cs ZE H	(18) LfxEto Cs E H
MDR TB	(6–9) Km LfxEto Cs ZE (modify treatment based on the level of INH resistance as per the footnote)	(18) LfxEto Cs E

Note: All MDR-TB isolates would be subjected to LC DST at baseline for Kanamycin and Levofloxacin, the results of which would be received after 6–8 weeks. Appropriate modifications of the treatment regimens can be done in the presence of additional resistance.

XDR TB

XDR TB cases will be treated with the STR (standard treatment regimen) for XDR TB comprising of Injection Capreomycin, Moxifloxacin, Linezolid, PAS, Clofazimine high dose INH and Co-amoxyclav.

The duration of IP will be for 6–12 months. Only the injectables will be stopped in CP and the remaining medicines will continue for Another 18 months in CP.

All DR-TB treatment regimen are to be given on daily basis under supervision.

Daily regimen for XDRTB		
Type of TB case	Treatment regimen in IP	Treatment regimen CP
XDR	(6–12) Cm, PAS, Mfx, High dose-H, Cfz, Lzd, Amx/Clv	(18) PAS, Mfx, High dose-H, Cfz, Lzd, Amx/Clv

RATIONALE OF SWITCH OVER TO DAILY REGIMEN

High relapse rate of 11–13% has been reported in patients treated by DOTS intermittent regimen in the RNTCP in India from several different locations, over the last several years. In India isonex resistance is 11% in untreated TB patients and 37% in previously treated cases and the prevalence of HIV Co-infection is 5%. In countries where H (isonex) resistance is prevalent a full 6 months course of rifampicin is recommended with a third drug, Ethambutol, added to the 4 months continuation phase which is also safe in paediatric patients. Based on the above evidences and to have uniformity of care across healthcare sectors, universal access to quality TB care and prevention of further drug resistance to TB the choice of daily regimen using FDC (Fixed dose combination) under direct observation is required in India. The concept of daily, directly observed therapy (DOT) incorporating a full 6 months of R (Rifampicin) has been adopted by the majority of countries worldwide as a major part of **Stop TB Strategy**.

DOTS PLUS STRATEGY

It includes all the five components of RNTCP. DOTS plus is a strategy for management of drug resistant TB; (DR TB).

The treatment of DR TB is much more complex and lengthy in comparison to treatment of drug sensitive TB and requires special care to manage adverse drug reactions. DRTB patients are treated primarily on ambulatory basis after a brief period of in-patient care at initiation of treatment. The facilities for initiating of treatment are designated as DRTB **centres** and are normed at 1 per 10 million population across country. A linked DRTB centre is decentralized clinical unit under DRTB centre which provides treatment services to stabilized patient of DRTB. Currently there are 136 DRTB centres supported by 50 linked DRTB centres. DRTB diagnosis and sensitivity test are supported by 64 RNTCP certified culture and drug sensitivity laboratories in the country. 25 laboratories in the country are certified for second line DST (SLDT) laboratories, 6 National reference labs and several intermediate reference laboratories have been set up.

- 121 Cartridge Based Nucleic Acid Amplification Test (CBNAAT) provide rapid decentralized diagnosis of MDR–TB, TB in high risk group, PLHIV and paediatric presumptive TB.

TREATMENT OUTCOMES FOR DRUG-SUSCEPTIBLE TB PATIENTS

Cured: Microbiologically confirmed TB patients at the beginning of treatment who was smear or culture negative at the end of the complete treatment.

Treatment completed: A TB patient who completed treatment without evidence of failure or clinical deterioration BUT with no record to show that the smear or culture result of biological specimen in the last month of treatment was negative, either because test was not done or because result is unavailable.

Treatment success: TB patients either cured or treatment completed are accounted in treatment success.

Failure: A TB patient whose biological specimen is positive by smear or culture at the end of treatment.

Failure to respond: A case of paediatric TB who fails to have microbiological conversion to negative status or fails to respond clinically/or deteriorates after 12 weeks of compliant intensive phase shall be deemed to have failed response provided alternative diagnoses/reasons for non-response have been ruled out.

Lost to follow up: A TB patient whose treatment was interrupted for 1 consecutive month or more.

Not evaluated: A TB patient for whom no treatment outcome is assigned. This includes former "transfer-out".

Treatment regimen changed: A TB patient who is on first line regimen and has been diagnosed as having DRTB and switched to drug resistant TB regimen prior to being declared as failed.

Died: A patient who has died during the course of anti-TB treatment.

New Initiatives

1. Single window service delivery for TB and HIV with CBNAAT, fixed dose combination daily therapy(FDC).
2. Introduction of daily regimen for treatment of drug sensitive TB under RNTCP in 104 destricts of five states and now scaled up in whole of India in November 2017.
3. Scaling up of cartridge based nucleic acid amplification test (CBNAAT) machines in all districts.
4. Baseline second line anti TB drug susceptibility testing (SLDT).
5. Introduction of Newer Anti-TB drug **Bedaquiline** to improve outcome among drug resistant TB patients with drug susceptibility testing (DST) guided treatment.
6. Active case finding programme in vulnerable populations and geographical areas.
7. ICT enabled adherence support system to HIV TB Patients at all ART centres in India (99 DOTS). Patient makes a call every day to the revealed toll free number from any phone to report their adherence to daily drug regimen.
8. *Notification and surveillance*: TB disease was made notifiable disease in 2012. NIKSHAY Platform is being used under RNTCP as an ICT enabled state of art surveillance system to get notification of TB cases at diagnosis from both public and private sector including drug resistant TB patients.
9. National Tuberculosis Prevalence survey in 2018.

Engaging Private Sector in RNTCP

The private sector is predominant provider of health care service delivery in India. As per National Sample Survey Organization report of 71st round of survey more than 70% of patient seek care in private sector. Private sector accounts for almost 50% of TB care in India. This sector is unregulated and provides variable quality of services. Private practitioners may not **follow standards** for TB care in India, may over-depend on X-rays may not adhere to duration of treatment, etc.

Therefore engaging private sector effectively is the **single most important intervention** required for India to achieve the overall goal of universal access to quality TB care. RNTCP extends public services to private sector, involves them as partners, supplies free drugs and diagnostics involves them in notification-NIKSHAY and provides short term training courses.

Medical colleges involvement: Most medical colleges have been involved in the programme for specialist services, training programme and research activities besides advocacy programme.

International Standards for TB Care (ISTC)

RNTCP and World Health Organization Jointly prepared 26 standards for TB care in India (STCI) in 2014 to improve quality of services and management.[18-20]

Standards for testing and screening for pulmonary TB, treatment regimen follow up and monitoring and laboratories have been formulated and being implemented in the programme (RNTCP) by states. Private sector must adopt these standards of care.

Achievements of RNTCP

- Treatment success rate have tripled from 25 to 87%.
- High cure rate of over 87% has been achieved, thus TB is a curable disease.
- Mortality due to TB has declined
- Prevalence levels have come down.
- TB services are universally accessible covering total population.
- Standards for TB care in India have been adopted to provide high quality services.

Problems/Challenges

1. The decline of TB incidence is slow.
2. Emergence of Drug resistant TB has become a major public health problem.
3. Engaging private sector effectively.
4. Active case detection.

References

21. GOI, MOH and FW Revised National TB control programme-technical and operational guidelines for tuberculosis control in India 2016.
22. National Urban Health Mission—RNTCP collaborative Activity framework for implementation of urban slum intervention in Haryana March 2017.
23. WHO country office for India Standards for TB care in India 2014.

NATIONAL LEPROSY ERADICATION PROGRAMME (NLEP)

National Leprosy Control Programme was launched in 1955 and national Leprosy Eradication programme launched in 1983. Prevalence of leprosy in India was very high at 57.6 cases per 10000 population in 1981.

GOAL

To eliminate leprosy in the country by 2018. Elimination means less than 1 case per 10000 population in all the districts. India achieved leprosy elimination at National level in December 2005 as prevalence level of leprosy declined to 0.84 cases per 10000 with multi drug therapy (MDT).

Programme Components

i. Case detection and management

ii. Disability prevention and medical rehabilitation

iii. Information eduction and communication and behaviour change communication.

Epidemiological Situation

Though the prevalence level of less than 1 case per 10000 population has been achieved at, **National Level**, however 163 **districts** and many blocks of various states have prevalence level higher than 1 case per 10000 population. It has been observed that annual new case detection rate (ANCDR) and prevalence rate (PR) are almost static since 2006 (Fig. 12.3) and percentage of grade II disability increased from 3.10% in 2011 to 4.61% in 2015. High disability rate indicates delayed reporting and large number of cases still undetected in the community. In view of these observations activities for leprosy case detection were intensified by launching special drive in **high endemic districts** (163 districts).

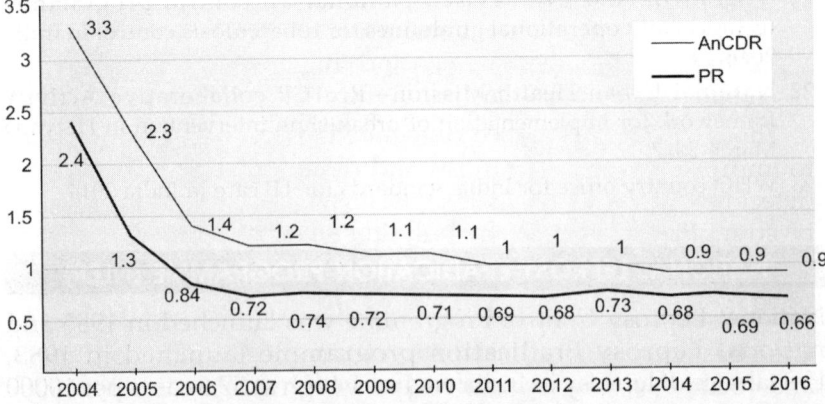

Fig. 12.3: Leprosy prevalence and new case detection rate per 10000 population

Leprosy Case Detection Campaign (LCDC)

a. LCDC in line with pulse polio campaign was initiated in 163 high endemic districts of 20 states to achieve the goal of elimination. House to house visits by team consisting of ASHA and male volunteer (Field level worker) as per microplan for block and district level for case detection, were undertaken. House to house activities were supervised by field supervisors. Case detection campaign was followed by treatment of all 32666 new cases detected in 400 million population.

b. **Strengthen disability prevention and medical rehabilitation in leprosy:** More emphasis is being given on correction of disability in leprosy affected persons through reconstructive surgery (RCS). Besides government NGOs institutions were also involved in RCS.

c. **Reduction in the level of stigma associated with leprosy:** Intensive information, education and communication activities are being conducted for awareness generation to reduce stigma and discrimination against leprosy affected patients. 30th January of every year is being observed as Anti-leprosy day.

d. **New initiative in 2016–17:** Chemoprophylaxis with single dose–rifampicin for contacts of new leprosy cases during leprosy case detection campaign and on line reporting of leprosy cases have now begun.

   Mycobacterium Indicus Pranii (MIP) vaccine developed in India can be given to people living in close contact of new cases, to be given along with dose of rifampicin. It is being pilot tested in 5 districts of Bihar and Gujarat.

e. **SPARSH leprosy campaign:** For spreading awareness about the disease and stigma reduction is being conducted all over the country involving gram sabhas. Inter-sectoral coordination between various sectors such as Panchayati Raj Institutions, Rural and Urban development, women and child development and social Justice and empowerment is being attempted to reduce stigma.

Though the NLEP has been integrated with general health services to improve access to diagnosis and treatment, the system fails to detect new cases. LCDC is a partial answer. Health system need to be strengthened by capacity building and regular monitoring.

FROM MALARIA CONTROL TO MALARIA—ELIMINATION

Case based and focus based surveillance: In malaria case based and **focus based investigation** has been initiated under malaria elimination programme since August 2017.

National strategic plan (2017–30) for malaria elimination has been launched in 2017.

Elimination–Definition: Zero indigenous case of malaria in the entire country by 2027. Maintain zero incidence and prevent reintroduction of malaria after elimination till 2030 and beyond.

All the states have been classified into 4 categories based on API

- **Category 0:** Prevention of **re-establishment phase** (states and UTs with zero indigenous case of malaria).

- **Category 1: Elimination phase** (states and UTs including their districts reporting an API of less than 1 case per 1000 population at risk.

- **Category 2: Pre-elimination phase** (states and UTs with an API of less than 1 case per 1000 population at risk, but some of their districts are reporting an API of 1 per 1000 or above).

- **Category 3:** States/UTs with an API of 1 case or more than 1 case per 1000 population at risk. All Districts, CHCs, PHCs, SCs and sections should be classified into above mentioned categories based on the annual parasite incidence (API) as the main criteria. District is a unit under malaria elimination programme.

Surveillance in Category 3 (Intensified Control Phase)

ACD—Active Case Detection

ACD is carried out by trained health workers (MPHW/ANM) with bi-valent antigen detecting RDTs through fortnightly house to house visits to cover 5000 population in plain and 3000 in tribal/hilly areas.

PCD—Passive Case Detection

- By trained health volunteers (ASHA, USHA, CHV) at community level and at **subcentre** by ANM with bivalent antigen detecting RDTs.

- At PHC/CHC/District hospital/Medical collage and private practitioners/dispensary, etc. the PCD is done through microscopy only, however bivalent antigen detecting RDTs will be used in emergent situations, odd hours, and non availability of Lab. technician results of microscopy should be made available within 24 hours.

- If a fever case is found positive for malaria, treatment should be initiated within 24 hours of detection and ensure complete treatment.

Referral system should be in place to deal with severe cases of malaria to prevent deaths

• Surveillance should sustain monthly blood examination rate (MBER) of minimum 1.5% during transmission months.

Surveillance in Category 2 (Pre-elimination Phase)

Same as category 3 given above. In addition more focused attention in project areas and construction sites and among migrant populations and slum population.

The monthly blood examination rate (MBER) should be sustained at a minimum of 1% during transmission months.

Case based and Focus Based Surveillance in Category 1 (Elimination Phase)

• Malaria should be made notifiable.
• ACD will be carried over by trained community level health workers (MPHW/ANM) by house to house fortnightly visits and collecting blood smears for microscopy examination*.
• PCD will be carried out by trained community level health volunteers/health workers—ANM at subcentre, dispensary PHC, CHC, District hospitals and Medical colleges and private and other sectors by blood smear collection for microscopic examination*.

*If a fever case is found to be positive for malaria. It should be **notified** and following actions should also be taken:*

i. **Prompt treatment:** Initiate treatment within 24 hours of detection and ensure complete treatment.
ii. **Case investigation:** Detailed case investigations are carried out and a case is classified as indigenous or imported, introduced, induced or relapsed case. Case investigations should be completed within 3 days of detection.
iii. **Contact survey:** Should be carried out by blood smears collection for microscopy in the surrounding 50 households by ASHA/MPHW/Technical supervisor.
iv. If additional cases are found on contact survey the area should be expanded and appropriate action initiated within 7 days.
v. **Follow up:** Positive case should be followed up to ensure completion of treatment.

---

*However bivalent antigen detecting RDTs will be used in areas where microscopy results are not available within 24 hours, in emergent situations and odd hours when microscopy facility is not available.

vi. The annual blood examination rate (ABER) should be sustained at minimum of 7% in perennial transmission and minimum 5% in seasonal transmission areas.

Case Based and Focus Surveillance in Category 0 (Prevention of Re-establishment Phase)

- Malaria should be made notifiable.
- Any fever case reporting to a health care provider/facility (private and others) and meets the case definition of suspected malaria (intermittent fever with rigors and sweating in a high endemic area) should be investigated using microscopy examination of blood smear.
- If a case is found positive for malaria it should be immediately notified to authorities and the actions I–VI as elaborated in elimination phase above should also be taken.

Screening at the points of entry at International and inter-state borders should be established for the purpose of cross reporting, enumeration of cases and public health action.

Case based surveillance in malaria: Every case of malaria is reported and investigated immediately and also included in the weekly reporting system. Each confirmed case of malaria in category zero and 1 requires both detailed epidemiological **case** and **focus** investigation by rapid response teams. **Each** case and focus is investigated and classified.

Case Investigation

Collection of information to allow classification of malaria case by origin of infection, i.e. whether it was imported, introduced, indigenous, induced or relapsing. Case investigation may include administration of standard questionaire to a person in whom malaria infection is diagnosed as well as screening and testing of people living in the same household and surrounding areas of 50 households.

Indigenous Case

A case contracted malaria locally with no evidence of being imported or being directly linked to transmission from an imported case.

Imported Case

Malaria case or infection in which the infection was acquired outside the area in which it is diagnosed.

Induced Case

A case whose origin can be traced to blood transfusion or other form of parenteral inoculation of parasite.

Introduced Case

A case contracted locally, with strong epidemiological evidence linking it directly to known imported case.

Relapsing case: Recurrence of asexual parasitaemia in P. vivax or P. ovale infections. Relapse occurs when hypnozoites persist in liver and mature to schizonts which after an interval of 3 weeks to one year rupture and release merozoites into blood stream.

Focus Investigation (Geographical Reconnaissance)

Once a case of locally acquired malaria has been detected, the second stage of surveillance, i.e. focus investigation is carried out to describe the area where malaria occurred and delineate the population at risk. A **malaria focus** is **defined** as a **circumscribed area** in a currently or former malarious area that **contains** the **epidemiological** and **eco'ogical** factors necessary for malaria transmission such as breeding places, mosquito density, anophelese vectors, human behaviour, e.g. sleeping outdoors and occupation, and to decide or choose appropriate intervention. The focus is classified into-active, cleared up, potential and pseudo focus.

1. **Pseudo-focus:** Where conditions are not suitable for malaria transmission throughout the year.
2. **Active focus:** Where there is an evidence of current transmission or history of recent transmission, e.g. during the past two years and presence of introduced and/or indigenous cases.
3. **Cleared up focus:** No case is present in the circumscribed area.
4. **Potential focus:** It is a focus where only imported or induced or relapsing cases are present.

Epidemic Response

Early detection and early response to malaria outbreak is essential in all categories of malaria elimination, however it is most critical in prevention of re-establishment phase, as even a single case of malaria during this phase has a potential of focal outbreak.

Malaria vaccine: WHO has recently announced that the World's first malaria vaccine to be rolled out through pilot project in three countries of Sub-Saharan Africa in 2018. The vaccine is known as RTSS against P. falciparum. It provides partial protection against malaria in young children.

NEGLECTED TROPICAL DISEASES (NTDs)

NTDs are a group of diverse communicable diseases that prevail in tropical and sub-tropical conditions in 149 countrie and affect more than a billion of people. These diseases mainly affect poor people living in insanitary conditions in close contact with infectious vectors and domestic animals and livestock. Many of these diseases can be eliminated by effective interventions. List of 18 NTDs is as under:

- Buruli ulcer
- Chagas disease
- Dengue and chikungunia
- Guinea worm disease
- Echinococcosis
- Foodborne trematodiases
- Sleeping sickness
- Leishmaniasis
- Leprosy
- Lymphatic filariasis
- Onchocerciasis
- Rabies
- Schistosomiasis
- Soil transmitted helminthiases
- Taeniasis/cysticercosis
- Trachoma
- Yaws
- Mycetoma

In India National Control/elimination programmes against NTDs have been launched. Yaws and, guinea worm disease have been eliminated successfully. National Programmes of Control of Rabies, National Deworming programme, elimination of lymphatic filarias, leprosy elimination, trachoma control National blindness control, National vector borne disease control programme, Kala Azar elimination programmes are under way in India.

Neglected Tropical Diseases

i. National Filaria Elimination Programme—Page 492.
ii. National Kala-azar Elimination Programme—Page 495
iii. Dengue/dengue haemorrhagic fever (Fig. 12.4)—Outbreak prone disease–with killer instinct—Page 497.

Recent Advance in Dengue

Dengue vaccine: At present no licenced vaccine is available in India. Dengue vaccine (Dengvaccia) has been licensed in Mexico, Brazil, Philipines, and EI Salvador. It is a live recombinant tetravalent vaccine. Recommended for age group 9–45 years. Three injection schedule spread over one year—0, 6 months and 12 months. Its efficacy is low—60%. It would be as an adjunct to other preventive measures against vectors such as rapid and effective larval source reduction by environmental modification and manipulation and measures against adult vector by space spray during outbreaks.

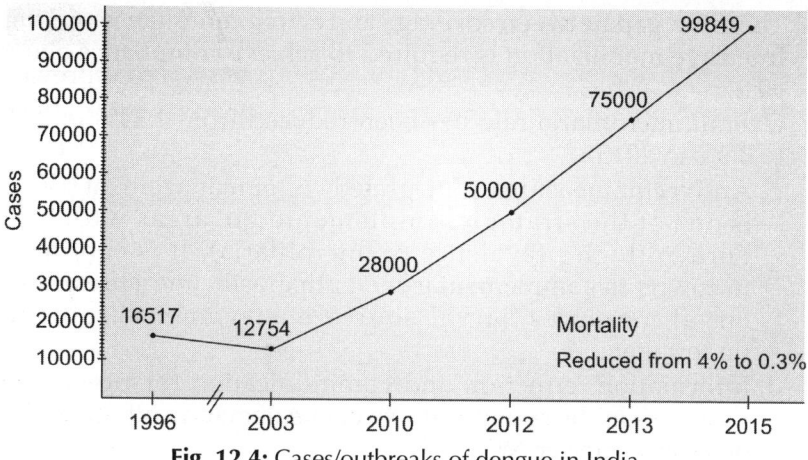

Fig. 12.4: Cases/outbreaks of dengue in India

- National Rabies Control Programme—Page 537
- National Deworming Programme—Page 169
- Hydatid Disease, Taenia and Cysticercosis—Page 550 and 551.

ELIMINATION OF LYMPHATIC FILARIASIS

Goal: Global goal is to eliminate lymphatic filariasis by 2020. National Health Policy 2017 advocates elimination by 2017/2018.

What is Elimination?

Achieving microfilaria rate of less than 1% in children of 6–7 years old in all the districts as a unit of elimination.

Strategy for Elimination of Lymphatic Filariasis
Supervised Annual Mass Drug Administration (MDA)

Initially the MDA was done with single drug DEC, since 2007 co-administration of DEC + Albendazole was introduced for MDA.

  a. Single dose of DEC (Diethylcarbamazine) and Albendazole for minimum of 5 years or more to whole of population at risk except pregnant women and children below 2 years of age and seriously ill persons to interrupt transmission of disease.
  b. Home based management of lymphoedema cases and up-scaling of hydrocele operations in identified CHCs/districts hospitals/medical colleges.

Coverage levels of MDT and reduction of disease:

- Reported coverage levels have improved from 73% in 2004 to 89% in 2015.

- There is a **gap between** coverage and actual compliance of drug. Intensive mobilization is required to achieve compliance above 90%.
- Overall microfilaria rate has been reduced from 1.24% in 2004 to 0.3% in 2015.

  c. **Antivector measures**—Integrated vector management (IVM)- is one of the strategies implemented in areas with high burden (high prevalence of microfilaria). It is continued in towns as complementary to antiparasitic measures. Anti-larval measures/larval source management are being undertaken.
  d. Information, eduction and communication for preventive measures in the community, to create demand and utilization of services under NFEP.

Transmission Assessment Surveys—For Monitoring and Evaluation

Phasing out of MDA has been started through validation. The validation is done through transmission assessment surveys (TAS). The TAS is a decision making tool for stopping MDA in a district (Fig. 12.5).

As per WHO guidelines of 2011 if a district having observed minimum five rounds of MDA or more, and achieved coverage level of more than 65% of population at risk in each round in the implementation unit (population of district covered under MDA) are subjected to transmission assessment surveys. TAS uses immunochromatographic test (ICT) for presence of circulating

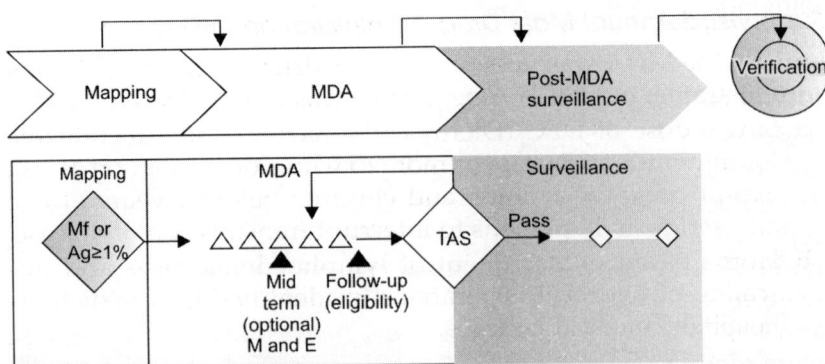

Fig. 12.5: Steps for interrupting transmission of lymphatic filariasis by mass drug administration (MDA) as described by WHO in 2011. TAS—Transmission assessment survey; M and E—Monitoring and evaluation; Mf—Microfilaria

antigenemia/microfilaraemia. If the current infection rate is less than 1% in children 6–7 years of age (born after initiation of MDA) the area passes for TAS and MDA is stopped. Thus TAS is required to take a decision for MDA stoppage. As of now, 94 districts out of 256 districts have successfully completed or passed TAS and qualified for MDA stoppage.

All such districts which have successfully completed TAS are put under post MDA surveillance.

New Initiatives

* Study on triple drug (DEC + Albendazole + Ivermectin) therapy for MDA in Yadgir district of Karnataka.
* Introduction of DEC medicated salt as an adjunct to the existing MDA strategy.

JAPANESE ENCEPHALITIS (JE)—ACUTE ENCEPHALITIS SYNDROME (AES)

Japanese encephalitis (JE) is a mosquito borne zoonotic viral disease of public health importance because of its epidemic potential and high case fatality rate of 25% in children. In children who survive 30–40% may suffer from neurological sequelae-physical and mental impairment. The children suffer highest attack rate. The JE virus affects central nervous system.

Global Distribution

First discovered in 1924 in Japan as Japanese Encephalitis and now it is called JE. It is worldwide distributed-in Nepal, Bangladesh, Bhutan, China, Republic of Korea, Pakistan, Sri-lanka and Thailand.

Indian Scenario

It is endemic in 171 districts of 22 states. The states of Assam, Bihar, UP, Tamil Nadu and West Bengal are worst affected states. Over 375 million population in these states is at risk of JE. Epidemics are reported most often from UP and other northern states. Worst outbreak occurred in UP in 1986 when 7500 cases and 2627 deaths were reported. Thereafter in the year 2005 more than 6000 cases and 1500 deaths were reported. Over 11100 cases and 1289 deaths were reported in the year 2016 in India[2-6]. Outbreaks are common in areas where there is close interaction between pigs/birds and human beings. In 2017 many deaths due to JE were reported from Gorakhpur and Farukhabad in UP.

Causative Organism

It is caused by JE virus which belongs to genus flavivirus within the same genus are also present dengue virus, KFD, yellow fever and West Nile virus.

Reservoir

Primarily the JE virus circulates and multiplies in pigs and birds. In nature the virus of JE is maintained in Birds, Pigs and other animals. Pigs are major vertebrate hosts of JE.

Pig to pig cycle—it is maintained by culex vishnui mosquitoes. Pigs develop viraemia but donot manifest any sign and symptoms. Pigs and birds act as amplifying host in the transmission cycle.

Birds cycle—Ardeola grayii (pond heron) and Bubulcus ibis (cattle egret) play definite role in maintenance of virus in nature

Cycle: Pig ⇆ PiG ⇆ Birds
↓
Man—is dead end of transmission. Man to Man transmission not known.

Rural Urban Distribution

In India most of the cases and outbreaks over 90% occur in rural areas. These outbreaks have been associated with monsoon and paddy cultivation and piggaries close to households. The disease shows a scattered distribution of 1–2 cases reported per village. However JF/AES cases have also been reported from urban areas as well. For each clinical case in community there are 250 to 1000 inapparent infections. The cases of JE represent tip of the iceberg.

Trigger level: For JE is two cases of fever with altered consciousness/seizures in a village of 1000 population.

Man: Man is involved in the cycle incidently when mosquito density increases after rains and floods, the virus is transmitted from pigs to man by culex vishnui group of mosquitoes.

Vector: Culex vishnui group of mosquitoes (culex tritaeniorhynchus) are most important in transmission of JE virus from pigs to man. **Man** to **man** transmission is unknown hence man is the dead end of transmission of JE. The vector is exophilic (outdoor-resting habits after blood meal), hence indoor residual spray (IRS) not helpful. Vector breeds profusely in paddy fields and polluted water.

Incubation period—in man is 5–14 days. The extrinsic incubation period in mosquito is 9–12 days.

Age and Sex and Case Fatality Rate

JE affects vast majority of children below 15 years of age. Case fatality rate (CFR): CFR in children is very high at 25%. Those children who survive, 30–40% develop neurological sequelae like mental impairment, personality changes and paralysis.

NATIONAL PROGRAMME FOR PREVENTION AND CONTROL OF JAPANESE ENCEPHALITIS/ACUTE ENCEPHALITIS SYNDROME (AES)

In view of the evidence of the **entero-viruses** and **other non JE viruses** circulating in the endemic areas of Eastern Uttar Pradesh and occurrence of cases of JE round the year, the Government of India, on the recommendations of Group of ministers, launched National Programme for prevention and control of JE/AES in 2014. The National Programme of JE covers 60 high priority districts in the states of Assam, Bihar, Uttar Pradesh, West Bengal and Tamil Nadu.

Goal

The goal of the programme is to reduce morbidity, mortality and disability in children due to JE/AES.

Objectives

i. To strengthen and expand the programme of JE vaccination in affected districts.
ii. To strengthen surveillance, vector control, case management and timely referral of serious and complicated cases.
iii. To increase access to safe drinking water and sanitation in rural areas and some urban areas.
iv. To estimate disability burden due to JE/AES and to provide for adequate facilities for physical, medical, neurological and social rehabilitation.
v. To improve nutritional status of children at risk of JE/AES.
vi. To carry out intensive IEC/BCC activities.

Strategies or Interventions[7-11]

Convergence of Ministries

Convergence of different ministries at various levels is the **core strategy** for prevention and control of JE/AES. Nodal ministry or department of health and family welfare is responsible for expansion of JE vaccine, case management, surveillance, monitoring and evaluation besides IEC and behaviour change communication activities and physical rehabilitation.

Ministry of drinking water and sanitation is responsible for provision of safe drinking water and sanitation in rural areas, in view of risk of transmission of AES through contaminated water by enteroviruses. Ministry of housing and urban povery alleviation for safe water and sanitation in urban slums, Ministry of social justice and empowerment for establishing departments of physical and medical rehabilitation in medical colleges and district rehabilitation centres for disabled and Ministry of human resource development for arranging special facilities for eduction of disabled and Ministry of women and child development for improvement of nutritional status of children in affected areas through ICDS programme. Thus multipronged strategy for prevention and control of JE/AES has been evolved and it is big challenge to coordinate all the activities at ground level implementation.

STRENGTHENING AND EXPANSION OF JE VACCINE PROGRAMME

JE vaccine (SA-14-14-2) for all children 1-15 years of age in campaign mode, in endemic areas were launched in 2006. After that JE vaccine became part of universal immunization programme. Now all young children in endemic areas get two doses of JE vaccine first dose at 9 months and second at the age of 16-24 months under routine immunization programme since 2013. The programme has been expanded to cover 198 districts of endemic areas of JE.

- **Adult JE vaccination:** All adults between 15 and 65 years of age get one dose of JE vaccine in selected high burden districts of JE.

STRENGTHENING PUBLIC HEALTH ACTIVITIES

Additional resources in terms of manpower and material have been provided to endemic states, for containment of JE/AES.

- **District model action plans**—have been developed for community based surveillance, entomological surveillance, vector control and IEC/BCC activities.

JE/AES—SURVEILLANCE

The purpose of JE surveillance is: Early detection of outbreaks, estimate disease burden, geographical spread, disease pattern, incidence and trends over the years for prevention and control of JE as also programme evaluation.

SURVEILLANCE MECHANISMS

For surveillance purposes JE is commonly reported under the heading of "Acute encephalitis syndrome–AES". In the WHO guidelines for JE surveillance syndromic surveillance for JE is recommended. This means all cases of AES should be reported. The following case definition should be used for reporting of suspected JE cases in endemic areas:

Case Definition of Suspected Case

- Acute onset of fever, not more than 5–7 days duration.
- Change in mental status with or without:
    - New onset of seizures (excluding febrile seizures)
    - Other early clinical findings—may include irritability somnolence or abnormal behaviour greater than that seen with usual febrile illness

Important

- In an endemic situation fever with altered sensorium persisting for more than 2 hours with a focal seizure or paralysis of any part of body is **encephalitis**.
- Presence of rash on body excludes JE.
- AES with symmetrical signs and fever is likely to be cerebral malaria.

Laboratory confirmation of suspected cases can be done where feasible, e.g.

a. Sentinel surveillance sites with laboratory services at district level (SSSL)

b. Sentinel surveillance sites (SSS) without laboratory services– linked to **laboratory** services.

c. Informer units (IU)—smaller health facilities or private practitioners.

d. Routine reports of IDSP—for syndromic surveillance of JE.

JE Oubreak Investigations and Management

Surveillance data analysis gives information for predicting outbreaks of JE. Rapid Response team should start immediate containment measures after investigations. Control measures include–vector control by malathion fogging in the affected village, use bed nets and other personal protective measures and effective case management and eduction of community.

All cases that are notified should be verified and investigated by designated surveillance medical officer/epidemiologist within 48 hours of notification to confirm that case meets case definition and collect serum or CSF for lab test.

BETTER CLINICAL MANAGEMENT OF JE/AES CASES

As there is no specific treatment, JE patients require more supportive therapy such as feeding, maintain airways, anticonvulsants for seizure control and management of intracranial pressure which requires close monitoring. Under the programme 10 beded paediatric intensive care units (PICUs) have been set up at district hospitals of 60 priority districts for management of critical cases.

VECTOR CONTROL

JE vectors are exophilic (outdoor resting habits after blood meal) and endophagic in nature. The risk of transmission increases when the human dwellings and animal sheds particularly piggeries are situated very close to each other. Because of outdoor resting habits of vector using indoor residual spray is technically not appropriate. Due to vast and enormous breeding habitats like perennial ponds, paddy fields and other water bodies, larval control using various anti-larval measures are not feasible as it is resource intensive. Therefore vector control using ultra low volume (ULV) fogging with malathion/pyrethrum is the only method for vector control and can be used during JE epidemics also.

Setting up of Department of Physical Medicine and Rehabilitation (PMR) at Medical Colleges and Disability Rehabilitation Centres at District Level

In view of residual neurological sequelae in 30–40% of children who recover from JE/AES there is 'felt need' of rehabilitation centres for assessment and management of disabilities/

impairments. Departments of PMR in 10 medical colleges have been set up in endemic areas besides district disability rehabilitation centres in 60 districts. District counselling centres have also been set up in endemic areas.

Information Education and Communication and Behaviour Change Communication

The prime objective of IEC is to inform and educate people on all aspects of JE to increase demand for available services under JE and utilization of these services promptly. The second objective is to enhance community participation in all the programme components and interventions by using multi-media channels of communication.

Monitoring Supervision and Coordination

Monitoring reports are collected on daily basis during outbreaks/epidemic, weekly basis during transmission period and once a month during the inter-epidemic period. Based on the monitoring indicators, feed back and corrective actions are ensured at various levels to reduce morbidity, mortality and disability due to JE.

INTENSIFIED DIARRHOEA CONTROL FORTNIGHT (IDCF)

Childhood diarrhoeal diseases continue to be a major killer among under-five children in many states contributing to 12 percent of under-five deaths in the country. Almost all the deaths due to diarrhoea can be averted by preventing and treating dehydration by use of Oral Rehydration Solution (ORS) and administration of zinc tablets along with adequate nutritional intake by the child with diarrhoea. Diarrhoea can be prevented with safe drinking water, hand-washing, sanitation, immunization and breastfeeding/appropriate nutrition.

To combat diarrheal mortality in children with the ultimate aim of zero child deaths due to childhood diarrhoea, Intensified Diarrhoea Control Fortnight (IDCF) is being implemented as a campaign in the month of July, since 2014 for control of deaths due to diarrhoea across all states and UTs. It includes awareness generation on use of ORS and zinc during diarrhoea, bringing together multiple departments and also to reach each under-five child with one packet of ORS to be used when diarrhoea begins. Main activities include intensification of advocacy activities, awareness generation activities, diarrhoea management service provision, establishing ORS-zinc demonstration sites, ORS distribution by ASHA, detection of undernourished children and their treatment, promotion of Infant and Young Child Feeding practices (IYCF) by home visits by ASHA and establishing IYCF corners.

From 11–23 July, 2016, with an aim of achieving improved coverage of essential life-saving commodity of ORS, zinc dispersible tablets and appropriate child feeding practices during diarrhea, ORS was pre-positioned in houses of 5.4 crore children (provisional data), and 3.8 lakh ORS-Zinc corners were established. However sustained activities for prevention and control of diarrhoea at household and community level are essential which requires behavior change and effective response by mother/ parents.

Measles Elimination and Control of Rubella/Congenital Rubella Syndrome

Government of India along with 10 SEAR countries resolved to eliminate measles and control rubella/congenital rubella syndrome by 2020.

Measles-Rubella (MR) Campaign

Measles and rubella (MR) also contribute significantly to India's child mortality and morbidity. MR vaccine protects against measles as well as rubella. A wide age range MR campaign targeting children aged 9 months up to 15 years of age is to be conducted in phased manner over a period of 2–3 years. Subsequently a rubella vaccine will be introduced as MR vaccine in routine immunization as two doses replacing the currently measles vaccine 1 and 2 given at 9–12 months and 16–24 months respectively.

Coverage Evaluation Surveys on Immunization

NFHS-4 2015–16 Indicate that

i. 62% of children 12–23 months of age were fully immunized (BCG, measles and 3 doses each of polio, DPT). BCG coverage was very high at 91.9%, Three doses of polio vacc: ne-72.8%, DPT 78.4% and Hepatitis B 62.8%, measles 81%, a id nearly 91% of children received vaccination from Governmé nt facility.

ii. Rapid survey on children (RSOC) 2013–14 indicated 65.2% of children fully immunized. Coverage of measles vaccine was 78.8% and 74.7% received 3 doses of DPT vaccine.

Global report on antibiotic resistance: Showed high rate of antimicrobial resistance (AMR). Based on AMR surveillance data of ICMR 2016 it was evident that over 50% of antibiotics use in hospitals being inappropriate. The ICMR has issued antimicrobial treatment guidelines for 10 common infections/syndromes—acute undifferentiated fevers in adults, antibiotic associated diarrhoea, device associated infections, infections in organ transplant, obstetric and gynaecology related infections, patients with severe sepsis, septic shock in ICUs, upper respiratory tract infections and urinary tract infections.

ZIKA VIRUS DISEASE

What is ZIKA?

ZIKA is caused by a virus and transmitted by aedes mosquitoes, which is also the vector for dengue. In May 2015 Brazil reported first case of ZIKA, since then the disease has spread to 84 countries. The disease is commanding worldwide attention because of an alarming link with severe birth defect (microcephaly) and Guillain-Barré Syndrome. Babies born to infected pregnant women can develop **microcephaly**.

Common Symptoms

People with ZIKA can have mild fever, skin rash, conjunctivitis, muscle and joint pains, malaise or headache; symptoms last for 2–7 days.

Prevention

ZIKA can be prevented by preventing mosquito bites, source control-control breeding of aedes mosquitoes. No vaccine or specific medicine is available for disease. ZIKA is mild and requires no specific treatment. Treatment is symptomatic.

SPREAD

ZIKA virus out-break was declared by WHO as a Global Public Health Emergency of International Concern (PHEIC) on Feb 1, 2016. About 3 million cases were estimated in Latin American countries, hardest hit was Brazil with 1.5 million cases. PHEIC was declared as over in November 2016. ZIKA virus is a serious threat to health and well being of pregnant women and newborn child.

The World Health Organization (WHO) announced Zika virus outbreak in India in May 2017. Three laboratory confirmed cases from Ahmedabad in Gujarat were reported to WHO. Following this health ministry has decided to screen newborns with head circumference less than 31 cm for Zika related microcephaly. Their blood will be subjected to testing to rule out/confirm virus at 55 top institutes of the country.

WHO has not imposed any travel or trade restrictions as it was low level of transmission. WHO has asked the countries of South East Asia Region to take decisive steps to prevent, detect and respond to ZIKA virus.

INACTIVATED POLIO VACCINE-FRACTIONAL DOSE (FIPV)

Role of IPV (Table 12.2)

Adding IPV to the routine immunization schedule provides an immunity base to reduce the risk of polio disease in case any exposure to type 2 poliovirus following the switch from trivalent to bivalent oral polio vaccine (tOPV to BOPV). IPV and OPV work together to provide the best protection against polio.

What is **Fractional dose** IPV (fIPV)?

A fractional dose of IPV is a smaller dose of the same vaccine equal to 1/5 of a standard dose. Studies show that 2 doses of fractional dose IPV administered by **intradermal injection** produce an even stronger immune response than a single full IPV dose.

Fractional IPV should be given at the same time as the first and third doses of oral polio vaccine (OPV 1 and OPV3) drops, along with Penta 1 and Penta 3, at 6 and 14 weeks.

Intradermal dose is 1/5 of standard dose = 0.1 ml. Administer fIPV in the upper arm (opposite to that in which the BCG was given.

Two fractional doses of IPV given intradermally produce even better immunogenicity than a single standard dose (intramuscular).

Rotavirus Vaccine In UIP (Table 12.2)

Rotavirus vaccine is a live attenuated, oral liquid vaccine and is available in 10 dose vial and does not require reconstitution. The vaccine is in a liquid frozen form; In liquid form, the vaccine is generally pink in colour and may sometimes change to orange or light yellow in colour. The vaccine is supplied with pink colou ̄ed dropper.

Vaccination Schedule, Dosage and Route of Administration

The rotavirus vaccine is administered in 3 doses at 6, 10 and 14 weeks along with other UIP vaccines. NO booster dose of rotavirus vaccine is recommended.

Table 12.2: National immunisation schedule under UIP in India for pregnant women, infants, children and adolescents

Vaccine	When to give	Dose	Route	Site
For pregnant women				
TT-1	Early in pregnancy	0.5 ml	Intramuscular	Upper arm
TT-2	4 weeks after TT-1*	0.5 ml	Intramuscular	Upper arm
TT-Booster	If received 2 TT doses in a pregnancy within the last 3 years	0.5 ml	Intramuscular	Upper arm
For infants				
BCG	At birth or as early as possible till one year of age	(0.05 ml) 0.1 ml	Unitl 1 month Intradermal	Left upper arm
Hepatitis B (birth dose)	At birth or within 24 hours	0.5 ml	Intramuscular	Antero-lateral side of mid-thigh
OPV (zero dose)	At birth or within 15 days	2 drops	Oral	Oral
OPV 1, 2 and 3	At 6, 10 and 14 weeks	2 drops	Oral	Oral
IPV one dose	At 14 weeks with OPV3	0.5 ml	Intramuscular	Right mid thigh
DPT 1, 2, and 3	At 6, 10 and 14 weeks	0.5 ml	Intramuscular	Antero-lateral side of mid-thigh
Hepatitis B 1, 2, and 3	Do	0.5 ml	Intramuscular	Anterolateral side of mid-thigh
Rotavirus 1, 2 and 3	At 6, 10 and 14 weeks	5 drops	Oral	Oral

(Contd...)

Table 12.2: National immunisation schedule under UIP in India for pregnant women, infants, children and adolescents *(Contd...)*

Vaccine	When to give	Dose	Route	Site
Pentavalent 1, 2 and 3**	At 6, 10 and 14 weeks	0.5 ml	Intramuscular	Mid-thigh
PCV***	At 6 and 14 weeks	0.5 ml	Do	Do
Measles 1st dose	9 completed months–12 months	0.5 ml	Subcutaneous	Right upper arm
PCV booster	At 9 months	0.5 ml	Intramuscular	Mid-thigh
Vitamin A 1st dose	Do	1 ml	Oral	Oral
JE 1st dose****	9 completed months	0.5 ml	Subcutaneous	Left upper arm
For children and adolescents				
DPT 1st booster	16–24 months	0.5 ml	Intra-muscular	Anterolateral side of mid-thigh
OPV booster	16–24 months	2 drops	Oral	Oral
Measles 2nd dose	16–24 months	0.5 ml	Subcutaneous	Right upper arm
JE 2nd dose	16–24 months with DPT/OPV booster	0.5 ml	Subcutaneous	Left upper arm
DPT 2nd booster	5–6 yeasrs	0.5 ml	Intra-muscular	Upper arm
TT	10 years and 16 years	0.5 ml	intra-muscular	Upper arm
Vitamin A	The 2nd to 9th doses of Vitamin A can be administered to children 1–5 years old during biannual rounds, in collaboration with ICDS (Dose 2 ml)			

* Give TT-2 or Booster doses before 36 weeks of pregnancy preferably one month before expected date of delivery. However, give these even if more than 36 weeks have passed. Give TT to a woman in labor, if she has not previously received TT.
** Pentavalent vaccine contain a combination of DPT, HepB and HiB. In the states where it has been introduced, it will replace DPT 1, 2 and 3 and Hepatitis B 1, 2 and 3. Hepatitis B birth dose and booster doses of DPT will continue as before. IPV (inactivated poliovirus vaccine) along with 3rd OPV. Fractional IPV (fIPV) at 6 and 14 weeks.
*** PCV pneumococal conjugate vaccine.
**** JE vaccine (SA 14–14–2) is given in select endemic districts, after the campaign is over in that district.

Dose: Each dose of rotavirus vaccine consists of 5 drops. It is to be given orally at 6, 10 and 14 weeks along with first, second and third dose of OPV and pentavalent vaccine.

Phasing in

During the initial period of rotavirus vaccine introduction, only the infants coming for the first dose of OPV and pentavalent vaccine will be administered rotavirus vaccine. These children will be given 2nd and 3rd doses in subsequent visits as per schedule. The **maximum upper age limit** for giving first dose of rotavirus vaccine is **one year**. If the child receives first dose by 12 months of age, two more doses of vaccine should be given with an interval of 4 weeks between two doses to complete the course.

Infants who are coming for their second and third dose of OPV and pentavalent, will complete the schedule with OPV and pentavalent vaccine only. **Rotavirus vaccine is not to be started with second or third dose of OPV and pentavalent vaccine.**

Rotavirus vaccine is safe but contraindicated in child with history of documented intussusception or abdominal surgery or intestinal malformation and known cases of immunodeficiency or allergy.

The vaccine vial once opened to be used within 4 hours of opening. Open vial policy is not applicable for rotavirus vaccine. Any AEFI should be notified.

Reference

GOI NHM operational guidelines. Introduction of rotavirus vaccine in UIP in India. Immunization division MOH and FW GOI December 2015.

ROTAVIRUS-DIARRHOEA AND ROTAVIRUS VACCINE IN UIP

Rotavirus belongs to the viral family Reoviridae, which was named as "rota" virus due to its wheel like shape as visible under electron microscope.

BURDEN OF ROTAVIRUS DIARRHOEA IN INDIA

Rotavirus is leading cause of severe and fatal diarrhoea in children under five years of age. In India 40% of children hospitalized for diarrhoea are infected with rotavirus. Rotavirus is responsible for nearly 450000 to 884000 hospitalizations, and 2000000 outpatient visits. An estimated 1,22000 to 1,53000 diarrhoeal deaths annually in children in India are due to rotavirus, majority of these deaths occur in children under two years of age. Rotavirus in highly contagious and resilient. Nearly every child is at risk of infection, regardless of location, hygiene practices, or access to safe drinking water or sanitation. There is no specific treatment currently available to treat rotavirus diarrhoea. The only specific protection is by immunization with rotavirus vaccine.

Mode of Transmission

Rotavirus is highly contagious. Individuals suffering rotavirus diarrhoea often shed large amounts of virus in the stool. Rotavirus spreads primarily by the faecal oral route directly from person to person or indirectly by contaminated fomites. Infection occur in early childhood period, by the second year, most children are exposed to rotavirus and develop protective antibody. Hence vaccine is to be given during infancy.

Prevention: Integrated Approach

Sanitation and hygiene improvements have less impact on transmission of rotavirus diarrhoea which is thought to be due to person to person contact. Rotavirus vaccine along with other preventive measures such as exclusive breastfeeding for 6 months, continued breastfeeding with complementary feeding, Vit. A supplementation, and management of diarrhoea with ORS and zinc for 14 days, safe drinking water, sanitation and Hygiene (WASH) will benefit and impact in reducing under five deaths due to diarrhoea.

Pneumococcal Conjugate Vaccine (PCV)

Pneumococcal pneumonia is responsible for an estimated 5.6 lakh cases and 1.05 lakh deaths in young children in India. Pneumococcal vaccine provides protection against pneumococcal pneumonia a major killer in children under five year age group. PCV has been introduced in select districts of five states of Himachal Pradesh, Bihar, Rajasthan, MP, and UP in may 2017 and gradually will be scaled up in other areas. PCV will be given in three doses schedule at 6 weeks, 14 weeks and booster dose at 9 months under universal immunization programme to prevent one lakh deaths due to pneumonia in children.

13 Epidemiology of Non-Communicable Diseases and Related National Health Programmes

MODIFIABLE RISK FACTORS OF CARDIOVASCULAR DISEASES (CVDs)

I. Tobacco Use

Tobacco use in any form is prevalent in 28.6 of adults is India Tobacco use is harmful to all the systems of the body and more so for heart. Tobacco use increases atherosclerosis, raises the level of cholestrol. Nearly 31% of cases of ischaemic heart disease are attributable to smoking and tobacco use. Nicotine—the main agent in tobacco is the most addictive substance and it causes increased heart rate, blood pressure and reduces oxygen supply to tissues by converting haemoglobin to carboxy-haemoglobin by carbon monoxide in tobacco smoke.

II. Physical Inactivity

The world health survey found that overall 29% of the population had inadequate physical activity. Overall physical inactivity was estimated to cause 3.2 million deaths. Globally physical inactivity is attributable to 20% ischaemic heart disease. At least 30 minutes of moderate intensity of physical activity on most of the weekdays is recommended for prevention of CVDs, 45 minutes for fitness and 60 minutes per day for weight reduction. Physical activity reduces the risk of IHD, diabetes, strokes, hypertension and depression.

III. Hypertension

Globally it is estimated that 62% of cerebrovascular disease and 49% of ischaemic heart disease are attributable to sub-optimal blood pressure. High BP increases the work of heart and produces hypertrophy of left ventricle. Increase in bulk of heart muscle means increased oxygen demand for heart muscle. Since at the same time blood flow is facing an obstruction the heart does not get enough oxygen. This is how the high blood pressure increases the risk of heart attacks. High BP also produces brain haemorrhages.

IV. High Level of Cholesterol—VLD Lipids and Triglycerides

Hypercholesterolaemia is a risk factor of CVDs (Coronary heart disease and stroke). Cholesterol is key component in the development of atherosclerosis—the accumulation of fatty deposits on the inner lining of the arteries. High cholesterol is estimated to cause 56% of global ischaemic heart disease and 18% of cerebro-vascular disease. Diets rich in saturated fats, sugar and salt causes high cholesterol levels. Fats and oils consumption is very high in urban households at 159% of adequacy (NIN survey 2017).

V. Diabetes Mellitus

Diabetes is a risk factor of CVD and is a leading cause of renal failure. Reduction in the risk of CVD with well controlled diabetes is well established but this requires a control of other risk factors too. Diabetes increases the risk of CVDs 2–3 times in men and 3–7 times in women.

VI. Obesity

Obesity itself is a risk factor for ischaemic heart disease, ischaemic stroke and type 2 DM, apart from many other conditions such as cancers, gall stones and joint problems. Nearly 58% of diabetes and 21% of ischaemic heart disease globally are attributable to BMI above 21 kg/m^2. Normal range of BMI for Indians is 18.5 to 22.9, overweight BMI is between 23 and 24.9 and obese grades of BMI is 25 and above. As per ICMR-NIN survey 2017, over 34% of men and 44% of women in urban areas were obese.

VII. Low Fruits and Vegetables Intake in India

Dietary surveys reveal that fruits and green leafy vegetables (GLV) consumption is low in Indians. Fruits and GLV are rich is dietary fibres, Vitamin C, β carotene, riboflavin, folic acid and anti-oxidants. These agents remove free radicals and lower the level of harmful cholestrol and promote the level of HDL–protective lipid as also prevent obesity and cancers of digestive system. Horticulture and agriculture policies can promote consumption of fresh fruits and

GLVs. Adequacy of consumption of GLVs was 59% in urban households.

VIII. Stress

Stress does exert adverse effects on heart and blood vessels. It results in release of hormones, which damage the inner lining of blood vessels. Such an injury promotes cholestrol deposition to produce atheroma. Stress hormones also damage the heart muscle and can change the properties of platelets and help in formation of clots. Avoid stress by Yoga and relaxation techniques.

IX. Harmful Consumption of Alcohol

Harmful consumption of alcohol along with saturated fats, free sugars, and refined carbohydrates leads to overweight and obesity.

PREVENTION OF CVDs

Preventive strategies against CVDs include, primordial, primary, secondary and tertiary prevention.

SURVEILLANCE OF RISK FACTORS OF CVDs

To achieve 25% reduction in mortality, epidemiological surveillance of risk factors is appropriate, to monitor trends, to evaluate risk reduction strategies and to improve the implementation of strategies in India[15]. Simple parameters such as weight, height, history of tobacco use, physical activity, diet and family history of CVD, etc. should be obtained periodically.

BMI NORMS FOR INDIAN POPULATION (Table 13.1)

Obese grades of BMI are on the increase and were prevallent to the extent of 20.7% in women against 18.6% in men. Malnutrition in adults (chronic energy deficiency) is on the decline and its prevalence in men and women was at 20.2 and 22.9% respectively. Thus India is facing the double burden of overnutrition and undernutrition in men and women and same is true in children.

Table 13.1: Nutritional status of men and women (obesity/overweight)				
	NFHS 3–200–06		NFHS 4–2015–16 figures in %	
	Men	Women	Men	Women
BMI < 18.5	34.2	35.5	20.2	22.9
BMI ⩾ 25	9.3	12.6	**18.6**	**20.7**

Norms for Indian population norms for BMI are as under:

Normal range of BMI	18.5 to 22.9
Overweight BMI	23 to 24.9
Obese grade BMI	More than 25

NON-COMMUNICABLE DISEASES (NCDs)

Over the last 26 years, the country's disease pattern has changed (Table 13.2). Disease burden due to most communicable, maternal, neonatal and nutritional problems has declined, at the same time the burden of Non-communicable diseases and injuries has increased and people live longer life now. There were large variations of disease burden in states and regions of the country.

Burden of NCDs in India in terms of mortality

Table 13.2: Trends of DALY loss (disease burden) by major disease groups from 1990 to 2016*

Major disease groups	Daly loss in percentages	
	Year 1990	Year 2016
I. Non communicable diseases	30.5	55.4
II. Communicable, maternal neonatal and nutritional	60.9	32.7
II. Injuries	8.6	11.9

* Source: Indian council of Medical Research, Public Health Foundation of India, and Institute for Health Metrics and Evaluation. India: Health of the Nation's States—The India State-Level disease burden initiative. New Delhi, India: ICMR, PHFI, and IHME; 2017.

NCDs were the leading cause of deaths in adults in India besides injuries, estimated to account for 60% of total deaths and cardiovascular diseases were number one killer among NCDs followed by chronic Resp. Diseases, Cancers and Diabetes (Fig. 13.1).

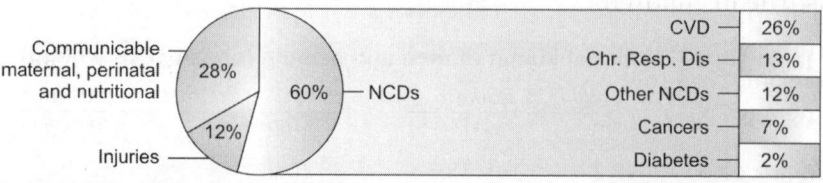

Fig. 13.1: Proportional Mortality due to non Communicable Disease in India 2014 (WHO 2014)

Global Burden of NCDs

A total of 57 million deaths occured worldwide during 2012, of these, 38 million were due to NCDs; principally cardiovascular diseases, cancers, and chronic respiratory diseases. Nearly three quarter of these (28 million) occured in low middle income countries (LMIC).

Burden of Non-communicable Diseases in India (Fig. 13.1)

Non communicable diseases (NCDs) are currently leading cause of preventable deaths and disability in India. The identified major NCDs are cardiovascular diseases—such as heart attacks and stroke, Hypertension, Obesity, Diabetes, Chronic Obstructive Pulmonary Diseases, Asthma, Cancer and Injuries. They are leading causes of death, accounting for over 60% of premature mortality placing them ahead of Communicable diseases, Maternal, Perinatal and Nutritional conditions (WHO 2014)[6]. As per study of **ICMR, PHF** and **IHME** 2017, the proportion of deaths from NCDs have increased from 37.9% in 1990 to 61.8% in 2016.

To address the problem of NCDs National Programme for Prevention and control of cancers, diabetes, cardiovascular diseases and strokes (NPCDCS) has been launched in 2010 after integrating the National Cancer Control Programme with NCDs.

NATIONAL PROGRAMME FOR PREVENTION AND CONTROL OF CANCER, DIABETES, CARDIOVASCULAR DISEASES AND STROKES (NPCDCS)

Components of NPCDCS

The programme has two components:

1. **Cancer prevention and control**
2. **Prevention and control of diabetes, CVDs and strokes.**

Global target of NCDs:

Premature mortality: (Sustainable Development Goals of UNs). The premature mortality target is a 25% reduction of overall mortality from cardiovascular diseases, cancers, diabetes and chronic respiratory diseases by 2025 (Referred to as 25 × 25) between the age 30 and 70 years from base year 2015.

Major objectives of NPCDCS:

i. To prevent and control NCDs (reduce morbidity and mortality).

ii. To provide early diagnosis and management of NCDs

iii. To build capacities at various levels.

Strategies/Interventions to Achieve the Objectives

i. Promotion of "healthy life styles" by education

ii. Specific protection

iii. Early detection by population based screening and opportunistic screening

iv. NCDs clinics at CHC and district level for management of NCDs

v. Development of trained manpower

vi. Strengthening of tertiary level facilities.

Major Risk Factors in NCDs (Fig. 13.2)

Most NCDs are strongly associated and causally linked with following major **Behavioural Risk Factors** (modifiable risk factors):

i. Tobacco use

ii. Physical inactivity

iii. Unhealthy diets—excessive consumption of fatty, sugary and salty foods.

iv. Harmful use of alcohol

v. Household air pollution

vi. Stress

Risk factors of NCDs are cumulative and operate on a life course perspective. All the behaviour risk factors are amenable to modification through life style changes. In nutshell today's risk factors are tomorrow's disease. The primordial, primary, secondary and tertiary prevention levels are the time tested approaches. Population based primordial and primary prevention are most valued and sustainable and best buy's in the long run, and much more cost effective. **Primordial prevention is real prevention.**

Non modifiable risk factors are—age, sex, heredity and family history. These are also associated with occurence of NCDs.

If the above behavioural risk factors are not managed or modified these can lead to Biological risk factors such as overweight/obesity, high blood pressure, raised blood sugar and raised level of total cholestrol or lipids. Disease outcome as a result of these risk factors are—CVDs, Cancers, COPD, and Diabetes (Fig. 13.2).

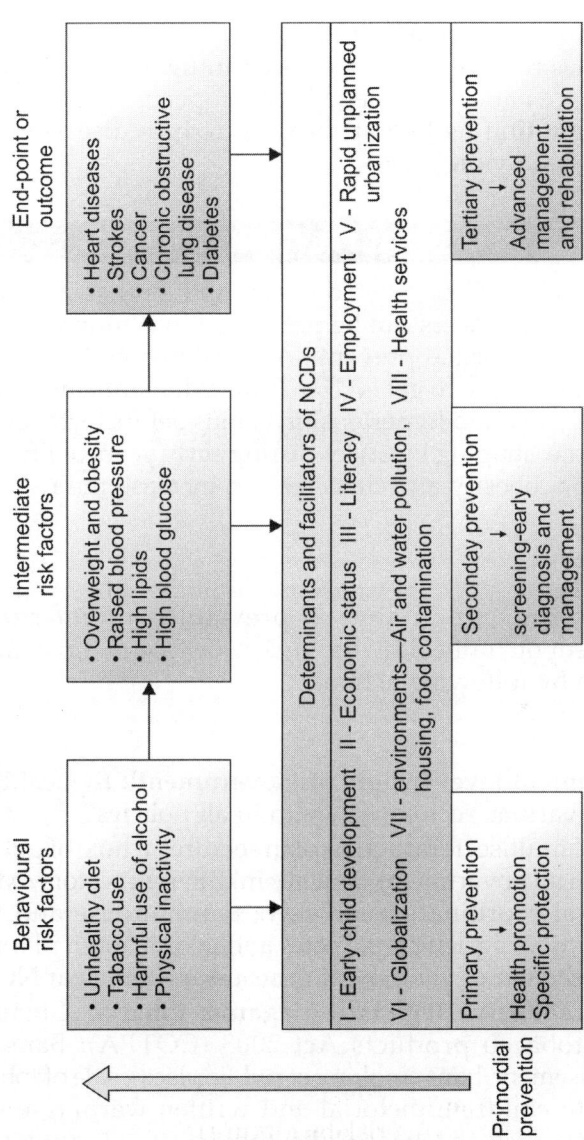

Fig. 13.2: NCDs risk factors and levels of prevention

The process of atherosclerosis starts at an early age. Most of behavioural risk factors begin during **early Childhood** period and adolescence and their effects appear in 4th or subsequent decades.

NCDs are very expensive to treat. Treatment is life long. Almost all the NCDs require continued care throughout the life span of a patient, hence national strategies have to focus on **prevention** and **health promotion** as **key strategy** to reduce disease burden by adopting Healthy life styles.

PRIMORDIAL PREVENTION IN NCDs

Approximately 80% of heart diseases and strokes, 80% of type 2 DM and 30% of cancers can be prevented by eliminating common risk factors. Primordial prevention is real prevention, which does not allow the people to get NCDs. Primordial prevention in CVDs, Diabetes, obesity and hypertension begins before birth and in early childhood, i.e. shaping lifestyles during early years of life. Maternal malnutrition, obesity and diabetes can increase the risk of NCDs in children.

AIM/GOAL

Primordial prevention aims at prevention of emergence and development of "unhealthy life styles" or "Known risk factors" in population by following actions:

Actions

At Government level (whole of Government): By healthy public policies in various sectors—"health in all policies".

National multisectoral action plan requires whole of government or 'health in all government' policies in different sectors/Ministries. Intersectoral coordination between health, excise and taxation, home, eduction, agriculture, youth and sports, town planning and women and child development is necessary to defeat NCDs.

  a. **Comprehensive legislation against tobacco:** Cigarette and other tobacco products Act 2003 (COTPA): Bans tobacco advertisement, bans smoking at public places, sale of tobacco products to children, pictorial and written warning on tobacco products such as tobacco kills, tobacco causes cancer.

   • Crop alternatives to tobacco-to curb-production of tobacco.

   • WHO framework convention on tobacco control (FCTC) has been adopted by India—a landmark in tobacco control.

b. **Agriculture and nutrition policy:**
  - Production and promotion of protective foods—green leafy vegetables and fruits, whole grain cereals and pulses and regulating their prices.
  - Healthy foods through mid-day meal programmes in schools and Anganwadis

c. **Food industries:** Regulating the salt content and trans fats in processed foods, ban on Junk foods or sin-tax (heavy tax on junk foods).

d. **Education and sports-youth:** Promoting physical activities–excercises and yoga in schools and work place and in colleges.

e. **Women child and development:** National nutrition policy—Food security and promoting traditional foods, improving infant and young child feeding practices (IYCFP).

f. Prevention of household air pollution by use of clean fuel/energy in kitchen. Govt gives subsidies on LPG to BPL families.

g. Town and country planning for parks and open spaces.

At Community Level, whole of Society by Health Education and Health Promotion

Prevention of emergence of risk factors of NCDs in population by adopting healthy lifestyles beginning from early childhood period, continued during adolescence and maintaining healthy lifestyles during rest of the life (lifecycle approach) are most appropriate. Begin communication and education on healthy living, healthy food habits during preschool period at home and at anganwadi centre, continued at schools, in colleges by teachers and peer groups, by employers at work place followed by active ageing. Family holds primary responsibility in shaping and development of healthy lifestyles in their offsprings. Multi-media approaches/multi sectoral approaches for education and communication be adopted for developing healthy lifestyles such as:

Healthy Foods/Healthy Diets

Eating habits get established during infancy and childhood period. Parents and school teachers hold key position to promote healthy eating habits.

- Avoid eating fast/junk foods and use of carbonated drinks.
- Increase intake of protective foods such as green leafy vegetables, fresh fruits and sprouts.
- Consume whole grain cereals, mixed cereals and pulses and seasonal vegetables.

- Avoid fatty-sugary and salty foods. Limit salt consumption to less than 5 g per day. Refined carbohydrates–maida, bread, etc. excess sugar, excess of saturated fats and fried foods increases the risk of NCDs particularly CVD and diabetes. Wholegrain cereals and pulses are good for health, these foods provide fibres and lower cholestrol levels.
- Use unsatuated fats or oils such as groundnut, soyabean and sesame oil and sunflower oil, and moderate consumption of Desi Ghee, vanaspati and animal fats. Vegetarian diets are safer and better. Excess eating of junk foods and use of carbonated drinks and refined carbohydrates (noodles, fried fingers, burgars, potato wafers, Sweets and samosa) can lead to overweight and obesity in children and adults.

Promote Physical Activities and Excercises at Home, Schools and Workplace

Promote physical activities and excercises right from early childhood period to avoid overweight and obesity. Regular excercise (moderate to vigorous) for 5–7 days per weak along with yoga and meditation by all can prevent obesity. At least 30 minutes of moderate intensity physical activity per day is good for heart to prevent CVD, 45 minutes per day to stay fit and 60 minutes per day for weight reduction along with healthy eating. Patients or sick should seek advice of their physician for excercise. Physical activity reduces the risk of coronary heart disease, type 2 diabetes, stroke, colon and breast cancers.

Weight Control—Obesity an Epidemic

Overweight and obesity is a disease in itself and a risk factor for CVDs, diabetes and hypertension and cancers (breast and colon). Weight control measures consist of eating sensibly and eating healthy foods and regular physical activities. Keep your BMI between 18.5 and 22.9. BMI between 23 and 24.9 is considered as overweight and BMI of 25 or more than that is obese grade BMI. Nearly 10% of rural and 25% of urban adults are obese. Nearly 25% of children in Urban areas are overweight and 10% are obese and hardly 20% of Delhi adolescents took on to any physical excercise (Anoop Misra).

Tobacco Use

Tobacco causes 1 million deaths in India per annum. It is a global killer. Tobacco use in any form is harmful to health. Tobacco use is a risk factor for development of CVDs, cancers, COPD, blood pressure and many other diseases. In India 28.6% adults and 4% of minors aged 15–17 years use tobacco and habit of use of tobacco begins during childhood/adolescent period. Education programmes in the community to develop smoke-free and tobacco free society can go a long way in primordial prevention. Parents in the family and school teachers are the role models for young children. Quiting smoking and tobacco use at any stage is beneficial for health, heart and lungs.

Avoid Harmful use of Alcohol

Alcohol consumption is a risk factor for oesophageal cancer, liver cancer and cirrhosis, stroke, homicide and motor vehicle accidents. By supply reduction and demand reduction in the community by education, and by legislative measures alcohol use can be controlled. Dependence and Harmful use of alcohol is prevalent in 4.6% of adults in India and in some areas it is much higher (Punjab, AP and Goa).

PRIMARY PREVENTION IN NCDs—BEHAVIOUR CHANGE COMMUNICATION

Once the risk factors or "unhealthy life styles" have been established or emerged in the population attempt is made to prevent the development of CVDs and other NCDs in persons having these risk factors. Purpose of primary prevention is to **limit** the **incidence** of NCDs in population by modification of known risk factors by **behaviour change communication**. There are two approaches in primary prevention of NCDs:

1. Population Based Approach II High-Risk Approach

I. *Population Based Approach or Interventions*

Population based approach focuses on risk factors reduction in whole population of infants, children, adolescent, youth and, reproductive age group and old people. Population based strategies for NCDs are much more beneficial, cost effective, sustainable and make high impact. Population wide behavioural risk factors modification and adoption of healthy life styles as norms for entire population: (such as "best buys advocated-by WHO" include tobacco control, dietary salt reduction, harmful use of alcohol, fats and sugar, physical inactivity and promoting hepatitis B vaccine and HPV vaccine, etc.) could prevent large proportion of NCDs in whole population. Moreover relationship between behavioural risk factors and development of NCD events is continuous and most

NCDs occur, in people, at middle range (or modest elevation) of multiple risk factors, who are not normally judged as high risk persons. Axiom—"a large number of people who are exposed to small risk may generate many more cases of NCDs than a small number or minority exposed to high risk" (Rose). Therefore reduce mean blood pressure of population, mean blood sugar levels, mean salt intake and mean cholestrol levels in population to ultimately reduce incidence and burden of NCDs by massive/aggressive health promotional activities for all in all age groups. Population based strategies that seek to shift the whole distribution of risk factors to the left have the potential to control population incidence. Population based approach does not require any screening programme.

Specific Protection by Immunization

HPV (Human papilloma virus vaccine) against prevention of cervical cancer is available. Bivalent HPV vaccines are effective and safe but these have been introduced in a few states. Hepatitis B vaccine prevents chronic hepatitis and liver cancer hence a "best buy". Protection against environmental risk factors for cancer such as aflatoxin, asbestos and contamination of drinking water can be effective prevention strategy. Tobacco control can prevent tobacco related cancers.

II. *High-Risk Approach—Screening of NCDs*

In the national strategy of control of NCDs more emphasis is on screening of individuals above 30 years of age for "Risk assessment" in this approach attempt is being made to screen out high risk individuals by **periodical medical check up** at regular intervals. Those individuals who show abnormal values are prescribed individualized programme directed at modifying or reducing or eliminating the risk factors and thus preventing CVDs and other NCDs in **minority of people**. Screening of risk factors is a costly affair. High risk approach benefits minority of people who are at risk of NCDs. The efforts expended on measuring risk factors in individuals, is therefore questionable (Robert Beaglehole). Screening for risk factors such as measuring blood pressure, glucose, waist circumference and BMI, overall check up cost time and lot of money hence a resource intensive activity. In contrast population based strategies that seek to shift the whole distribution of risk factors to left, have the potential to control population incidence by lowering the risk in the entire population.

Opportunistic Screening

Strategy for early detection of chronic NCDs consists of opportunistic screening of persons above the age of 30 years at the point of primary contact with any health care facility, be it a village, sub-centre, PHC, CHC, district or tertiary care hospital. Opportunistic screening identifies behavioural risk factors by history taking (Tobacco use, diets, physical activity, alcohol use, fuel use) and BP and glucose measurement. Opportunistic screening have in built component of mass awareness generation, self screening and screening by trained persons. Individual counseling and life style management and referral of high risks are other components of opportunistic screening programme.

Population-Based Screening for NCDs

Hypertension, diabetes and three common cancers (oral, breast and cervix).

Purpose of screening in NCDs is to identify risk factors, high risk persons and to detect a disease at preclinical stage or to detect syndrome at early stage. Screening focuses on apparently healthy people in target age group of 30–65 years. Screening is not a final diagnosis. Screening of risk factors or high risk persons is a costly affair. Screening must be supported with proven interventions and services close to the community. Screening of NCDs is an integral part of comprehensive primary health care at subcenter (health and Wellness Centre).

Focus: All men and women age group 30–65 years.

Frequency: Once a year for diabetes, hypertension and obesity in persons above 30 years.

Once in five years for oral, breast and cervix cancers in persons 30 to 65 years.

Who will screen: ASHAs, ANM under the supervision of LHV and medical officer and mid level provider. These workers are trained in oral visual examination, clinical breast examination, and visual inspection using acetic acid (VIA) for cervical cancer screening.

Population Enumeration

First step in the process of screening is active enumeration of population of persons over 30 years of age in each household/ family by ASHA; on individual health card. About 37% of persons in population are above 30 years of age.

Risk assessment screening: ASHAs will complete **community based assessment check** list (CBAC) of risk factors assessment by scoring system. Risk assessment includes questions on age, tobacco use, alcohol use, waist measurement, physical activity, family history of diabetes, hypertension and heart disease (Table 13.3).

A score above 4 indicates that a person may be at risk of NCDs and needs to be prioritized for attending weekly NCD day. A score below 4 implies low risk. Low risk score does not mean that individual is to be excluded from screening, as NCDs could exist even in the absence of risk factors. The scoring is not a point of elimination but a means to highlight risk factors. In addition, the tool includes questions related to symptoms for cancer cervix, breast and Oral cancers, epilepsy and COPD so that such cases can be identified and referred to appropriate centres. Screening for cervical cancer should take place at SC or PHC, i.e. at **health and wellness centres**.

If the symptoms of shortness of breath, coughing more than 2 weeks, blood in sputum, difficulty in opening of mouth ulcer/ patch/growth in the mouth that has not healed in two weeks, any change in tone of voice, lump in breast, blood stained discharge from the nipple, change in size and shape of breast, bleeding between periods, bleeding after menopause, bleeding after intercourse and foul smelling vaginal discharge are present the person is refered to medical officer of nearby facility. ANM undertakes blood pressure and glucose measurement and refers cases with high BP and blood glucose, and symptoms requiring investigations for cancer to appropriate facility for confirmation and initiation of treatment and follow up thereafter.

PART A—RISK ASSESSMENT—SCREENING BY ASHA

Table 13.3: Community based assessment checklist (CBAC) form for early detection of NCDs

Part A: Risk assessment		
Question	Range	Circle any Write score
1. What is your age? (in complete years)	30–39 years 40–49 years 50 years and above	0 1 2
2. Do you smoke or consume smokeless products such as Gutkha; or Khaini?	Never Used to consume in the past/ Sometimes now Daily	0 1 2

(Contd...)

Table 13.3: Community based assessment checklist (CBAC) form for early detection of NCDs *(Contd...)*

Part A: Risk assessment

Question	Range		Circle any Write score
3. Do you consume Alcohol daily?	No		0
	Yes		1
4. Measurement of waist (in cm)	Female	Male	
	<80 cm	<90 cm	0
	80–90 cm	90–100 cm	1
	>90 cm	>100 cm	2
5. Do you undertake any physical activities for minimum of 150 minutes in a week?	Less than 150 minutes in a week		1
	At least 150 minutes in a week		0
6. Do you have a family history (any one of your parents or siblings) of high blood pressure, diabetes and heart disease?	No		0
	Yes		2

Total score

A score above 4 indicates that the person may be at risk for these NCDs and needs to be prioritized for attending the weekly NCD day

Part B: Early detection: Ask if patient has any of these symptoms

B1: Women and Men	Yes/No	B2: Women only	Yes/No
Shortness of breath		Lump in the breast	
Coughing more than 2 weeks		Blood stained discharge from the nipple	
Blood in sputum		Change in shape and size of breast	
History of fits		Bleeding between periods	
Difficulty in opening mouth		Bleeding after menopause	
Ulcers/patch/growth in the mouth that has not healed in two weeks		Bleeding after intercourse	
Any change in the tone of your voice		Foul smelling vaginal discharge	

In case the individual answers Yes to any one of the above mentioned symptoms, refer the patient immediately to the nearest facility where a Medical Officer is available

Cancer Component of NCDs

The cancer control component of the programme has more than 27 regional cancer centres. The National Cancer Registry Programme has population based cancer registries to provide data on incidence, mortality rate and survival rates of cancers.

Burden: The international agency for research on cancer, the GLOBCAN project has predicted that the cancer burden due to oral, breast and cervical cancers in India will rise from one million cases in 2012 to over 1.5 million, i.e. 1569, 196 by 2035. Overall burden due to all cancer in India is 3.8 million cases (ICMR 2012).

Common cancers: The three most commonly occuring cancers in India are those of breast, uterine cervix and oral cavity. Together they account for approximately 34% of all cancers and hence public health priority in India. The odds of incurring catastrophic hospitalization expenditures are about 160% higher with cancer than communicable diseases.

Deaths: About 7 lakh deaths occur per annum in India due to cancers, most cancers, over 75 to 80% are detected late in advance stage when the prognosis and survival are poor. Screening programmes detect cancers at an early stage when the prognosis and survival is good. Five years survival rates for early stage cancers are as under:

	In early stage	*At late stage*
Oral cancers	60.2%	3.3%
Breast cancers	76.3%	14.9%
Cervical cancers	73.2%	7.9%

Warning Signals for Cancers

C—Change in bowl and bladder habits
A—A wound that does not heal
U—Unusual bleeding or discharge
T—Thickening or lump in the breast
I—Indigestion or difficulty in swallowing
O—Obvious change in wart or mole
N—Nagging cough or hoarseness of voice

CANCER—SCREENING OF COMMON CANCERS AND REFERRAL

Screening Methods

Cervical cancers: Visual inspection with acetic acid (VIA). 3–5% of acetic acid is applied on the lip of the cervix, a white patch developing after one minute of application indicates positive VIA test. The test can be performed by trained ANMs/Nurses/Doctors.

Breast cancer: It is the commonest cancer in women. Method of screening is clinical Breast examination by visual inspection and palpation. Self examination is best examination.

Oral cancer: Detection of pre-cancerous **lesions** in oral cavity such as leucoplakia and Erythroplakia by visual examination of oral cavity.

Inclusion criteria: Persons above the age of 30 years with periodicity of every five years. Self examination and reporting of any non healing lesion in oral cavity is best practice.

Secondary Prevention Against NCDs

This level of prevention applies to persons who have developed NCDs. Aim of secondary prevention is to reduce prevalence of NCDs in the community.

The Strategy of Secondary Prevention in NCDs
Early Diagnosis and Prompt Treatment

By opportunistic screening and population based screening for common NCDs and cancers.

Access to Affordable Treatment/Medicines (Table 13.4)

NCDs clinics have been set up at community health centres (CHCs) and district hospitals. The CHCs and district NCDs clinics provide comprehensive care and management of cardiovascular diseases, strokes, diabetes, hypertension, and common cancers (oral, breast and cervical cancers) in the OPD, and Indoor on all working days of the weak. CHCs and district hospitals have been strengthened by providing additional contractual staff and laboratory facilities. At the district level cardiac care unit with 2–4 beds has been set up. Cases from villages, subcentres, PHCs are referred to PHC, CHC and district for diagnosis and management and follow up.

Expected Outcomes

- The programme and interventions would establish a comprehensive sustainable system for reducing the rapid rise of NCDs, disabilities and deaths due to NCDs. Broadly, following outcomes are expected.
    - Reduction in exposure to risk factors, life style changes leading to reduction in NCDs
    - Improved quality of life

Table 13.4: Package of services for NCDs

Health facility	Packages of services
Sub centre	• Health promotion for behaviour change and counselling. 'Population based/Opportunistic' Screening of common NCDs including cancers (Breast cervix and oral) • Awareness generation of early warning signals of common cancers and other risk factors of NCDs • Referral of suspected cases to PHC/CHC/nearby health facility. Follow up of patient put on treatment
PHC	• Health promotion for behaviour change and counselling. 'Population based/Opportunistic' Screening of Diabetes, hypertension and three common cancers (oral, breast, and cervical by VIA) • Clinical diagnosis and treatment of common NCDs including Hypertension and Diabetes, referral of complicated cases of DM/HTN to CHC/DH. • Identification of early warning signals of common cancers • Referral of suspected cases to CHC/DH and follow up of patient put on treatment.
CHC/FRU	• Prevention and health promotion including counselling. Early diagnosis through clinical and laboratory investigation • Diagnostics facilities: Blood sugar, Total Cholesterol, Lipid Profile, Blood Urea, creatinine, X-ray, ECG, USG (To be outsourced, if not available) 'Opportunistic' screening of common cancers (Oral, Breast and Cervix) • Management of common NCDs • Referral of complicated cases to District Hospital/higher health care facility
District Hospital	• Diagnosis and management of cases of CVDs, diabetes, COPD, stroke and Cancer (outpatient, inpatient and intensive Care) including emergency services particularly for Myocardial Infarction and Stroke • Lab. investigations and Diagnostics: Blood sugar, Lipid Profile, KFT, LFT, X-ray, ECG, USG ECHO, CT Scan, MRI, etc. (To be outsourced, if not available) • Referral of complicated cases to higher health care facility. Health promotion for behaviour change and counselling. 'Opportunistic' Screening of NCDs including common cancers (Oral, Breast and Cervix) • Follow up chemotherapy in cancer cases, Rehabilitation and physiotherapy services

Table 13.4: Package of services for NCDs *(Contd...)*

Health facility	Packages of services
Medical College	• Mentoring of District Hospitals, Early diagnosis and management of Cancer, Diabetes, CVDs and other associated illnesses, Training of health personnel, Operational Research
Tertiary Cancer centre	• Mentoring of District Hospital and outreach activities, Comprehensive cancer care including prevention, early detection, diagnosis, treatment, palliative care and rehabilitation • Training of health personnel and • Operational research

– Early detection and timely treatment leading to increase in cure rate/control and survival
– Reduction in prevalence of physical disabilities including blindness and deafness.

Home based care: Bed ridden patients are provided home based care by nurses **available at CHCs**.

These clinics have been linked to tertiary cancer care centres of tertiary hospitals for advanced treatment. Apart from treatment these clinics undertake life style management and counselling services. Free diagnostics and drugs are supplied for treatment of NCDs.

Tertiary prevention in NCDs: This level consists of disability limitation and rehabilitation of advanced cases of NCDs. This level manages complications and sequelae of NCDs, like renal, retinal, strokes and haemorrhages, diabetic foot and palliative or terminal care in cancer. Rehabilitation consists of physical, emotional and psychological as also occupational rehabilitation. Home based and community based rehabilitation is a preferred strategy for NCDs.

The convergence and linkages with ongoing interventions of National Health Mission including National Tobacco Control Programme, National Mental Health Programme, National Programme for Health care of elderly, oral health and deafness prevention, RNTCP, adolescent/school health and RCH programme to achieve public health goals in an integrated manner by national multisectoral action plan.

Surveillance of Risk factors of NCDs: Regular, ongoing collection, compilation, analysis and interpretation of data on NCDs and their risk factors help to plan, monitor and evaluate the programmes of NCDs. It should be part of IDSP. Ten voluntary targets on NCDs can be Evaluated by periodic surveillance of risk factors of NCDs.

Multisectoral Action Plan for Prevention and Control of NCDs 2015

Vision: All Indians enjoy the highest attainable status of health and well being and quality of life at all ages, free of preventable NCDs, avoidable disability and premature deaths.

Goal: Reduce preventable morbidity, avoidable disability and premature mortality due to NCDs

Strategic Areas and Key Outcomes

- **Integrated multi sectoral coordination**—between eduction, agriculture, youth, and sports, food industries, town and country planning, transport and women and child welfare.
1. Establishment of plateform for multisectoral collaboration and attainment of health in all sectoral policies.

2. Health Promotion

Reduction of risk factors (Tobacco use, alcohol use, unhealthy diet physical inactivity in children and adults—Best Buy's).

3. Health System Strengthening

Ensuring NCDs health services under **universal health coverage**.

4. Surveillance, Monitoring and Research

Availability of timely information on progress on key indicators of monitoring network.

New Initiatives for Control and Prevention of NCDs

- Intervention for prevention and control of rheumatic heart disease (RHD) under NPCDCS and RBSK:
  - For prevention and control of RHD: Rashtriya Bal Swasthya Karyakram Teams would be used to generate awareness and screen suspected cases and refer them to nearest facility (DEIC)—district early intervention centre.
- Integration of AYUSH with NPCDCS:
  - Yoga as an intervention is being encouraged for prevention and management of common NCDs.
- Integration of RNTCP with diabetes as co-morbidity.

WHO Global Action Plan and Monitoring Framework for Prevention and Control of Non-communicable Diseases

The WHO Global action plan provides road map to attain ten voluntary global targets to be achieved by 2025 including 25 indicators for prevention and control of non-communicable diseases by a set of very cost effective interventions (Best Buys).

Targets

1. 25% relative reduction of premature mortality from cardiovascular diseases, cancer, diabetes and chronic respiratory diseases by 2025 (*Referred to as 25 × 25*).
2. At least 10% relative reduction in the harmful use of alcohol.
3. 10% relative reduction in prevalence of physical inactivity.
4. A 30% relative reduction of mean population intake of salt/sodium
5. A 30% relative reduction in prevalence of current tobacco use in person aged 15+ years.
6. A 25% relative reduction in the prevalence of raised blood pressure or contain the prevalence of raised blood pressure.
7. Halt the rise in diabetes and obesity.
8. At least 50% eligible people receive drug therapy and counselling (including glycaemic control) to prevent heart attacks and strokes.
9. An 80% availability of affordable basic technologies and essential medicines
10. Household indoor air pollution 50% relative reduction in household use of solid fuels as a primary source of energy for cooking.

NATIONAL MENTAL HEALTH SURVEY IN INDIA 2015–16

Burden of Mental Disorders in India

As per Global burden of disease report mental disorders account for 13% of total DALYs lost for years lived with disability, with depression being the leading cause.

> **ONE IN TEN INDIAN ADULT HAS SOME MENTAL DISORDER ONE IN 40 SUFFER FROM DEPRESSION (2.7%)**

OVERALL PREVALENCE

Prevalence of any mental disorder in adult Indian was 10.6% while life time prevalence rate was 13.7%. Translating to real numbers-150 million Indians are in need of active intervention/services.

a. **Common mental disorders (CMD):** CMD including depression, anxiety and substance use disorders are huge burden affecting nearly 10% of the population (Table 13.5).

Table 13.5: Prevalence of mental disorders in adults in India 2015–16

Description	Percentage
1. Any mental disorder	10.6
2. Common mental disorders (Depression, anxiety and substance use disorders	10.0
3. Severe mental disorders (Schizophrenia, Bipolar affective disorders and severe depression)	0.8
4. Substance use disorders	22.4
5. High suicidal risk	0.9

Source: National mental Health survey of India 2015–16

b. **Severe mental disorders (schizophrenia, BPAD and severe depression):** Affect nearly 0.8% of adult population. There is significant stigma, neglect and marginalization associated with these disorders as they affect all domains of life and require long term rehabilitation service.

c. **Substance use disorders:** Include harmful use of alcohol, moderate to severe dependance use of tobacco and illicit and prescription drugs which were prevalent in 22.4% of persons (Table 13.6).

d. Nearly 1% of population reported high suicidal risk in the past one moth. Suricide and suicidal ideation are important public health problems.

Suicide rate is one of the indicator of mental health status of a territory. In a limited study done in one rural community development block in Haryana, the proportion of suicidal deaths to total deaths was 6.67% and it ranked as 6th leading cause of mortality. It speaks of level of unrest, unemployment, unhappy married life and other social problems. Suicidal deaths were due to use of poisoning, predominantly celphos tablets

Table 13.6: Prevalence of tobacco use % 2010–17

Major drugs abused	Household surveys 2002	Mental health survey 2015–16
Tobacco	55.8	20.9
Alcohol	21.4	4.6
Cannabis	3.0	
Opiates	0.4	
Heroin	0.2	0.6
Other opiates	0.1	

(aluminium phosphide), burns, hanging and railway accidents, drowning, etc. Over 1.31 lakh suicide deaths are raported in 2013 (National Health Profile India 2016). WHO in 2012 reported 258075 suicidal deaths in India.

e. 7.3% children and adolescents (13–17 years age) have mental disorders translating to 9.8 million of young Indians. These disorders included depressive episodes, agoraphobia, intellectual disability, autism spectrum disorders and psychotic disorders.

f. **Intellectual disability** was prevalent in 0.6% resulting in 4 million persons requiring care.

g. **Epilepsy:** Prevalence of epilepsy was 0.3% or 2 million persons requiring care.

Significantly persons with mental disorders account for nearly a fourth of total case load in primary health care settings.

• 50% of those with mental disorders reported disability in all three domains of work.

Treatment Gap

Treatment gap of mental disorder ranged between 70 and 92% for different disorders. For common mental disorders treatment gap was to the extent of 85% while for severe mental disorders treatment gap was 73.6%

• National mental Health Survey data help to plan, implement monitor and evaluate the National Mental health programme.

MENTAL HEALTH CARE ACT (MHA) 2017

This Act replaces mental health Act of 1987.

AIM

The MHA aims to provide for mental health care for persons with mental illness and to protect, promote and fulfill the rights of such persons during delivery of mental health care.

It gives everyone an opportunity to write a will stating how they would like to be treated in case they contract mental illness in future—called "Advance directive". Institutional care (admission in hospital) cannot be against their will. Initial admission con not be more than 30 days. They have now right to appeal against their admission.

New Act says "Mental illness is a substancial disorder of thinking, mood, perception, orientation of memory that grossly impairs judgement, behaviour, capacity to recognize reality or ability to meet ordinary demands of life and mental conditions associated with abuse of alcohol and drugs. The Act does not include mental retardation".

Main Features of MHA

- Integration of mental health services with regular health systems.
- Provision of accessible, affordable and quality mental health services.
- Freedom to choose form of treatment and nominate a representative—a person, friend or relative.
- Protection from in-humane and degrading treatment.
- Not to be administered electric shock treatment (ECT) without anaesthesia and muscle relaxant; bans ECT in children.

Salient Changes in Policy on Mental Health

- Right based Act, it defines cruelty.
- Promotion of community based treatment.
- Special provision for women and children suffering from mental illness.
- Role of care givers recognized.
- Attempted suicide de-criminalized.
- It restricts psychosurgery.

GATS 2010 AND 2017

Table 13.7: Prevalence of tobacco use % 2010–17				
Users	Male	Female	All adults	
	2010	2010	2010	2017
Tobacco use in any form	47.9	20.3	**34.6**	**28.6**
Smokers	24.3	2.9	14.0	10.7
Users of smokeless tobacoo	32.9	18	25.9	21.4
Current cigarette smokers	10.3	0.8	5.7	4.0
Current bidi smokers	16.0	1.9	9.2	7.7

GATS 2016–17 revealed that the prevalence of tobacco use has decreased by 6% from 34.6% in GATS 1 in 2009–10 to 28.6% in GATS 2 in 2016–17 (Table 13.7).

As per report, over 62% adults thought of quitting smoking cigarettes, 54% thought quitting bidi and 46.0% adults thought of quitting smokeless tobacco because of warning on tobacco products.

These findings are consistent with the government's anti-tobacco policies, including the recent decision to have 85% of tobacco package area on both sides covered with pictorial warnings and a previous decision regarding pan India ban on gutkha.

Interestingly the prevalence of tobacco use among the younger population aged 15–24 years has reduced from 18.4% to 12.4% while the number of tobacco users has reduced by about 81 lakh in last seven years, tobacco products have also gradually become unaffordable. The average expenditure incurred on last purchase of cigarette, bidi and smokeless tobacco was Rs 30, Rs 12.5 and Rs 12.8 respectively. The expenditure on cigarette has tripled and that on bidi and smokeless tobacco has doubled since GATS-1, the survey found.

New Estimates of Blindness in India

Until now under national Programme of control of blindness in India, using a visual acuity cut-off of <6/60 in the better eye, the number of blinds estimated were 13 million in India.

Now India has adopted WHO criteria to define blindness. WHO defines blindness as "Inability to count fingers at a distance of 3 metres, i.e. visual acuity of less than 3/60 (Snellen) or its equivalent. Going by new definition the population of blind people in India will reduce to 8 million in 2017".

ELIMINATION OF TRACHOMA BY 2020

Global Trachoma mapping project has been initiated in 29 countries to eliminate trachoma by 2020.

Active trachoma prevalence in India has come down to 0.7% in children aged one to nine years much below the elimination target of less than 5% (WHO). Thus active trachoma in India stands eliminated awaiting WHO certification. However sequelae of trachoma are prevalent to the extent of 3.5 per 1000 persons above the age group 15 years, higher than WHO standards of 2 cases per 1000 people. India is commited to eliminate active trachoma and its sequelae by 2020. (The Tribune Chandigarh/Monday/ 11 December 2017 Aditi Tandon).

SAFE strategy for trachoma has been described on page 664.

Geriatrics—
"Add Life to the Years"

NATIONAL PROGRAMME FOR HEALTH CARE OF ELDERLY (NPHCE)

Longitudinal Ageing Study in India (LASI) project launched in March 2016. The LASI project has been initiated under tertiary level activities of the programme to assess the health status of the elderly (age 15–60 years) with a sample size of 60250, this project would be one of the largest comprehensive ageing surveys in the world. LASI project is conducted by IIPS (Deemed University), Mumbai in Collaboration with Harvard School of Public Health and Rand Corporation. The tertiary component of the programme has been renamed as **Rashtriya Varisht Jan Swasthya Yojna** (RVJSY).

The tertiary activities include, continuation of 8 Regional Geriatric centres and setting up of 12 New Regional Geriatric Centres, setting up of two national centres for ageing and special initiatives for 75+ population.

Health Management

COMPREHENSIVE PRIMARY HEALTH CARE (CPHC)

Comprehensive Primary Health Care (CPHC) is the path to **universal health care** in India. Pilot projects on CPHC were launched by states in 2015–16.

For CPHC the subcentres will be upgraded as **"Health and wellness centres"** and make it the first point of comprehensive primary health care. This level will provide **universal screening** to detect early symptoms of hypertension, diabetes and 3 common cancers (oral, breast and cervical cancers) apart from **basic primary health care services**. A mid level provider (a nurse or an AYUSH provider) would be trained in a six month bridge course by IGNOU. The frontline worker team of ASHA and ANM will be trained in team work and work **flow** management in primary health care. The referral support and training for CPHC will be provided by PHC, CHC and District hospital. This approach will create healthy India. Package of services for NCDs, CCD, and MCH will be integrated at the level of subcentre and upward; with National Health Mission.

HEALTH MANPOWER (HUMAN RESOURCES) IN HEALTH SECTOR IN INDIA-UP TO 2015

Human resources with suitable skill mix in health is most critical for delivery of health services to population, they consume 50 to 70% of health budget. Information on human resources available in government and private sector is incomplete.

There is acute shortages of specialists (over 80%) at the level of community health centres, similarly over 63% of multipurpose health workers males positions are vaccant and technical paramedics are in short supply. Manpower planning in health is critical to meet the health needs of people in rural and urban areas (Table 15.1).

Table 15.1: Health Manpower in India

	Numbers	Population ratio
Number of Allopathic registered doctors	960233	1:1305
Number of AYUSH registered doctors	744563	1:1684
Number of dentists	156391	1:8018
Registered ANMs	789796	–
Registered nurses and midwives	1,793,337	1:475
LHVs	56096	–
Pharmacists	673401	1:1875
ASHAs*	9.1 Lakhs	1:1000
VHNSC	5.1 Lakhs	1 per village

* Over 13.4 lakh honorary AWWs are available in rural and urban areas under ICDS programme at community level for women and child development.

SUSTAINABLE DEVELOPMENT GOALS (SDGs) VERSES MDGs

On 25th September 2015, the UN general assembly adopted the new development agenda "transforming our world—the 2030 agenda for sustainable development". The 17 goals of the new development agenda integrate all three dimensions of sustainable development (economic, social and environmental) around the themes of **people, planet, prosperity, peace** and **partnership** (5 Ps).

The SDGs seek to continue to prioritize the fight against poverty and hunger, while also focussing on human rights for all, and empowerment of women and girls as part of push to achieve gender equality. They also build upon, and extend, the MDGs in order to tackle the unfinished agenda/business of the MDGs era.

One of the 17 goals is to "ensure healthy lives and promote well-being for all at all ages". The health goal is associated with 13 targets including 4 means of implementation targets labelled as 3.a to 3.d. Overall the SDGs have 169 targets and 230 indicators. It car be noted that the MDGs on maternal mortality, child mortality a d infectious diseases have been retained in the SDGs framewo. k, augmented by new and more ambitious targets for 2030, and expanded to include neonatal mortality, and more infectious diseases such as hepatitis and water borne diseases. The targets on reproductive and sexual health care services and access to vaccines and medicines are also closely related to the MDG targets. The heart of SDGs is equity, which is founded on the concept of "Leaving no one behind", i.e. reduction of inequality within and among countries. MDGs were focused on mothers and children and people affected by HIV, TB and Malaria. In contrast the health SDGs address health and well being at all ages including newborn and children, adolescents, adult women and men and older persons (life cycle approach). SDGs also lay stress to achieve **universal health coverage** and reduce the burden of **non communicable diseases**.

MINISTRY OF HEALTH AND FAMILY WELFARE

The Union Ministry of Health and Family Welfare is instrumental and responsible for implementation of various programmes on a national scale in the area of health and family welfare, prevention and control of major communicable and non-communicable diseases, and promotion of traditional and indigenous systems of medicine. In addition, the ministry also assists states in preventing and controlling the spread of seasonal diseases, outbreaks and epidemics by providing technical assistance. Department of AIDS control has been merged with department of health and family welfare and is now known as National AIDS Control Organization (NACO). Department of AYUSH has been upgraded to Ministry of Ayurveda Yoga and Naturopathy, Unani Sidha and Homeopathy (AYUSH). Ministry of health and family welfare now comprises the following two departments each of which is headed by a secretary to the Government of India.

i. Department of health and family welfare (DHFW)
ii. Department of health research (DHR).

Directorate General of Health Services (DGHS) is an attached office of the department of health and family welfare and has subordinate offices spread all over the country. The DGHS renders the technical advice on all medical and public health matters and is involved in implementation of various health schemes.

ANMOL (ANM ON LINE)

Department of health and family welfare has developed a tablet based application called ANMOL. ANMOL acts as a job aid to the ANMs by providing readily available guidance based on RCH data entered. This standardizes the maternal and child care services provided by ANMs who are able to generate work plan. This ensures more prompt entry and updation of data as well as improvement in data quality, since the data is being entered "at source". Another important component of the ANMOL is audio video counselling to enhance awareness of beneficiaries. But ANMOL is no substitute for regular contacts with beneficiaries and involving them in work planning and participation in the programme. ANMOL is supported by UNICEF.

MONITORING AND SUPERVISION OF WORK PLAN OF SUBCENTRE

Monitoring of sub-centre services (Maternal Child Health and Family Welfare Services) mean periodic collection and analysis of selected **indicators** of health services. The process of monitoring helps the manager to determine whether key activities are being carried out as planned. An indicator could be simple count of events or services it could be, rate, ratio proportion or percentage.

"Service statistics in public health are numerical measurements of services rendered to individuals and to community through public health programme". This definition makes service statistics "a means to an end not an end in themselves".

Mere counts of what has been done are not very useful. The information collected through the service report should be linked to the population base, it is the **community that is the patient**.

In addition to selecting an **indicator**, the manager sets **performance standards** for each indicator. Actual performance is compared with planned performance (standard performance or "target".

Example:

$$\frac{\text{Number of outreach immunization sessions actually held per month} = 3}{\text{Number of outreach sessions planned per month} = 5}$$
result indicates that 60% of sessions were held and 40% missed

Another Example:

$$\frac{\text{Number of infants vaccinated in a month} = 4}{\text{Number of births occured in that month} = 10} \ 100$$
result indicates that 40% of infants were immunized against the target of 100%, there was a gap of 60% in coverage

Technique for Monitoring of Subcentre Services

Routine monthly-monitoring report (MMR)—of subcentre is an important tool for monitoring of activities at subcentre level as also the performance level of the health worker against the standard performance or planned performance. The gap between standard performance and actual performance and the root causes of the gap are determined for actions to improve performance of worker and subcentre. Besides MMR, direct observation at the site of service delivery, exit interviews, sample of households visit by supervisors, records analysis, and rapid surveys besides community monitoring can be other useful techniques of monitoring. Monitoring data accumulation help in evaluation of programme/institution/ service.

Health System Monitoring
Output Indicators (Service Utilization Indicators)
The services and goods/products produced as a result of health activities or health programme are outputs or immediate results. The most important types of outputs in primary health care are:

a. **Utilization** of the services

b. **Quality** of services provided

c. **Contacts** of those in need of or eligible for service and

d. **Access** to the service.

Utilization of Service
Awareness, availability, affordability, accessibility are major drivers of service utization.

- Acceptors/users, e.g. number or percent of under 3 year children enrolled for growth monitoring, number of outpatients, antenatals, deliveries conducted per month, condom, IFA tablets distributed per month, etc.
- Continuation, e.g. number or percent of active or current users of contraceptives.
- Number or percent of pregnant women given full course of iron and folic acid tablets.
- Government service utilization for curative services was low in rural and urban area (21–28%) respectively.

Quality of Care
- Number or percent of health workers using sterile needles and syringes for each immunization injection (one needle, one syringe one child).
- Number or percent of babies weighed correctly.

- Number or percent of women who receive correct information on immunization schedule.
- Counselling, e.g. number or percent of health workers who counsel mothers on nutrition needs of their children

Contacts

For example, number or percent of eligible couples contacted per month.

- Number or percent of households contacted by malaria workers.

Access to Service

- Physical distance, e.g. number or percent of population living within 5 km of health facility.
- *Time to reach a facility*: Number or percent of population who can reach subcenre within half an hour or PHC within an hour of travel or FRU within 2 hours of travel.

Most of the indicators are designed to be simple counts of activities or simple percentages. In many cases count will be sufficient. Ideally counts and percentages would be calculated. Poor quality of service can lead to drop outs and low service utilization, and poor knowledge, attitudes and practice.

Effects Indicators (Coverage Indicators)

Effects are changes in the knowledge attitudes, skills and behaviour or practice that result from the health service. **Behaviour** or **coverage** is a measure of proportion of the target group that is following a prescribed **behaviour** or **practice**.

  A. *Examples of practice*
    1. Proportion of eligible couples using modern contraceptives in India is 53.5%.
    2. Proportion of children under two years who are fully immunized in India was 62%.
    3. Proportion of mothers who initiate breast feeding within one hour of birth (42%)

  B. *Knowledge*: Proportion of women in reproductive age group who can name three methods of contraception.

  C. *Skills*: Percentage of mothers who can correctly prepare and administer ORS.

  D. *Attitudes*: Proportion of eligible couples in favour of spacing births/pregnancies.

SPENDING ON HEALTH CARE (Table 15.2)

Despite years of strong economic growth in India the total spending on healthcare in 2013–14 was about 4% of GDP. Global evidence on health spending shows that unless a country spends at least 5–6% of its GDP on health, and the major part of it is from Government expenditure, basic health care needs are seldom met. The Governement spending on healthcare in India is only 1.15% of GDP, i.e. less than 30% of total health spending. Perhaps the single most important policy pronouncement of the National Health Policy 2002 articulated in the 10th, 11th and 12th five year plans and the NRHM framework was the decision to increase public health expenditure to 2–3% of GDP. Public health expenditure rose briskly in the initial years of the NRHM, but at the peak of its performance it started stagnating at about 1.04% of GDP. The failure to attain minimum levels of public health expenditure remain the **single most important constraint.** While it is important to recognize the growth and potential of rapidly expanding private sector, international experience (as evidenced from the table below) shows that health outcomes and financial protection are closely related to absolute and relative levels of public health expenditure. Brazil, Thailand and Sri Lanka have achieved close to universal health coverage. Thailand has almost the same total health expenditure as India but its proportion of Public Health Spending is 77.7% of total expenditure, and this is spent through a form of strategic purchasing in which about 95% is purchased from Public Health Care facilities which is what gives it such a high efficiency. Brazil spends 9% of its GDP on health but of this public health expenditure constitute 4.1% of the GDP (45% of total health expenditure). It would be ambitious if India could aspire to public health expenditure of 4% of the GDP but national health policy of 2017 commits 2.5% of GDP on health as public health expenditure.

Table 15.2: Govt health spending on health in different countries			
Country	Total health exp. as % of GDP 2011	Govt health exp as % of total health exp 2011	Life expectioncy 2011
India	4.0	28.6%	68
Thailand	4.1	77.7%	75
Sri lanka	3.3	42.1%	75
Brazil	8.9	45.7%	74
USA	17.7	47.8%	79
UK	9.4	82.8%	81
Russia	6.1	59.8%	69

At such level of expenditure "purchasing" has to be mainly from public providers for efficient use of health resource with purchasing from private providers only for supplementation.

HEALTH CARE FINANCING IN INDIA AT A GLANCE

There were four major sources of health financing in India.

1. Household revenues for financing health care, 72.9%.
2. State Government Funds, 12.7%.
3. Central Government Funds, 7.8%.
4. Social Insurance, 6.0%.
5. Local bodies funds, 0.6%

High Out of Pocket Expenditure (OOPE)

Household revenues, which finances the **out of pocket** expenditures, is the single largest component (73% of current health expenditure). Out of which the out of pocket expenditure (OOPE) on health is estimated 64.2% of the total health expenditure and 69.1% of the current health expenditure (Fig. 15.1).

In India private expenditure nearly 73% of total expenditure on health is highest in the world, major burden of this falls on poor people, which results into catastrophic health expenditure. About 63 million people get impoverished every year on account of catastrophic health expenditure.

What is Catastrophic Health Expenditure?

Health care costs of a household exceeding 10% of total monthly consumption expenditure or 40% of its non food consumption

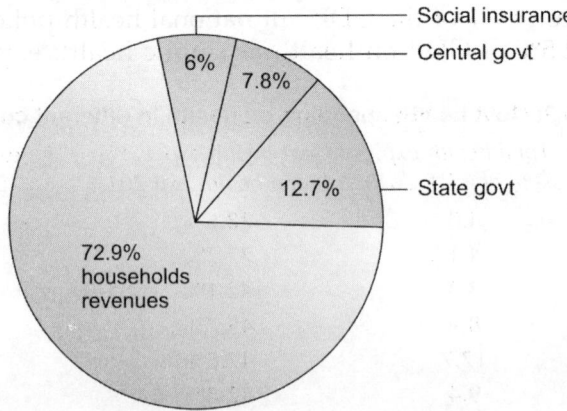

Fig. 15.1: Sources of Financing in India (NHA 2013–14)

expenditure is designated as **Catastrophic Health Expenditure** and is declared as an unacceptable level of health **care cost**. Impoverishment due to health care cost is of course even more unacceptable.

Private Health Sector

With 80% of doctors, 25% of nurses and 49% beds, private sector is dominant provider of curative services. This sector is financed primarily by out of packet expenditure (OOPE).

Major challenge of ailing Govt. Health sector is to increase its utilization in favour of poor. Health care utilization in India is predominantly through private sector for-curative care and towards government sector for preventive service. In fact more than 70% of spells of ailments were treated in private sector for the outpatient services. Similarly private institutions dominate in the field in treating inpatient from both rural and urban areas. About 58% of rural and 68% of urban people utilized inpatient services of private institutions. A steady decline in the of government sources and corresponding increase in the use of private sources over the last three NSS rounds was evident in urban areas. The changes were nominal in rural areas during the period between 2004 and 2014 (Tables 15.3 and 15.4).

Govt health sector is dominant provider of preventive and promotive health services to over 95% of the population of the country.

Health financing is critical for planning allocation of resources to develop strategies that protect people from catastrophic health expenditure and reduce inequities.

Table 15.3: Percentage distribution of spells of ailment treated during last 15 days by level of care separately

Level of care	Percentage of spells of ailment treated					
	Rural			Urban		
	Male	Female	Persons	Male	Female	Persons
1	2	3	4	5	6	7
SC, PHC and others*	10.6	12.3	11.5	3.5	4.2	3.9
Public hospital	15.9	17.5	16.8	17.4	17.3	17.3
Private doctor/clinic	52.7	48.9	**50.7**	48.9	50.8	**50.0**
Private hospital	20.8	21.3	**21.0**	30.2	27.7	**28.8**
All	100	100	100	100	100	100

Table 15.4: Percentage distribution of hospitalized cases by type of hospital (public and private) during 2014, 2004, and 1995–96: rural, urban

Type of hospital	Percentage of hospitalized cases in					
	Rural			Urban		
	1995–96	2004	2014	1995–96	2004	2014
1	2	3	4	5	6	7
Public	43.8	41.7	41.9	43.1	38.2	32.0
Private	56.2	48.3	**58.1**	56.9	61.8	**68.0**
All	100	100	100	100	100	100

State and Central Govt Revenues (Financed from General Taxation)

How Much we Spend on Health? Dismal Government Health Spending

The total health expenditure (THE) in both Government and private sectors providing health care in India during the financial year 2013–14 was estimated 4.02% of gross domestic product (GDP), which is broadly comparable to other developing countries at similar levels of per capita income. However the government expenditure on health (both central and state Govt) was dismal low at 1.15% of GDP which amounts to 28.6% of the total health expenditure; as a result 72.9% of health expenditure was in private sector and 64.2% being out of pocket expenditure of the total health expenditure. Total expenditure (private and government) in health per person per year was estimated at al Rs 3638, while government spent Rs 1042 per person per year. Govt revenues cater to 21–28% of outpatient care and 32–42% of inpatient hospital care in rural and urban areas respectively (Table 15.5).

Table 15.5: Expenditure on health in India 2004–05 to 2013–14

Selected National Health Accounts Indicators	2004–05	2013–14
1. Total expenditure on health as % of GDP	4.20	4.02
2. Public expenditure on health as % of GDP	**0.94**	**1.15**
3. General government expenditure on health as % of total expenditure on health	**22.5**	**28.6**
4. Private expenditure on health as % of total expenditure on health	78.05	72.9
5. Out of packet expenditure	69.4	64.2
6. Per capita public expenditure on health	₹242	1042
7. Per capita private expenditure on health	₹959	2596
8. Total per capita expenditure on health	120.1	3638

Source: World health Report 2007, NCMH-2005 and National health Accounts 2005 and 2013–14

According to National Health Accounts Estimates the Govt Health expenditure increased from 22.5 to 28.6% over the period of 10 years. Govt spends 51% of its health expenditure on primary health care, 23.3% on secondary and 13% on tertiary care. Only 9.6% of government expenditure is done on preventive care. Social health insurance expenditure as a share of total health expenditure increased form 4.2 to 6%. This has resulted to decrease in the out of pocket expenditure (OOPE) as a share of total health expenditure from 69.4% to 64.2% over the past 10 years.

Hospitalization Expenditure

a. **Average medical expenditure per hospitalization case:** On an average, a much higher amount was spent for treatment per hospitalized case by people in the **Private** (Rs 25850) than in **Public** (Rs 6120). The average medical expenditure for treatment per hospitalized case, if treated in private hospital was around 4 time than if treated in government hospital.

b. Average medical and other related non medical expenditure per hospitalization case in rural area was Rs 16956 against Rs 26455 in urban areas.

Strategic Purchasing of Secondary and Tertiary Care

Free primary health care by Government sector, supplemented by strategic purchase of secondary care hospitalization and tertiary care services from both public and private sector will be main financial strategy of assuring health services. Strategic purchasing means government acting as a single payer, purchasing care from private and govt hospitals for district health system development (NHP 2017).

Compulsory Social Insurance

Coverage of health insurance in India is pathetically limited. Compulsory social insurance schemes include the Central Government Health Scheme (CGHS), Employes State Insurance Scheme (ESIS), and Ex-service men Contributory Health Scheme (ECHS). Social health insurance expenditure has increased from 4.2 to 6% over the past 10 years.

Coverage of Health Expenditure Support (Social Insurance)

The Government was able to bring about 12% of urban and 13% of rural population under **health protection coverage** through Rashtriya Swasthya Bima Yojna (RSBY) or similar plan only 12% households of upper class of urban area had some arrangement of medical insurance from private providers. It is thus seen that as high as 86% of rural population and 82% of urban population were still not covered under any scheme of health expenditure support. On the whole poorer households appear not to recognize the efficacy of coverage, both in rural and urban areas.

A. Outpatient/Ambulatory Care Services (Fig. 15.2a)

It is observed that private doctors were the most important single source of treatment in both urban and rural areas. More than 70% (72% in rural and 79% in the urban areas) spells of ailment (outdoor care) were treated in the **private sector**—consisting of private doctors, nursing homes, private hospitals, charitable institutions. Only 28% in rural and 21% in the urban areas, spells of ailments were treated in **Government sector** consisting of Government hospitals, clinics, dispensaries, subcentres, primary health centres, community health centres, mobile medical units, ESI hospitals and dispensaries.

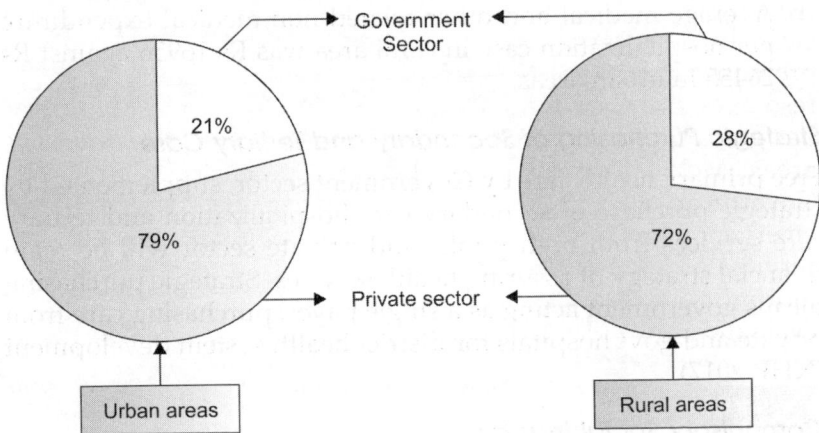

Fig. 15.2a: Percentage distribution of spells of ailments treated during the last 15 days in rural and urban areas by private sector and Government sector (NSSO 2015)

B. Inpatient/Hospitalized Care Services

Private institutions dominate in the field in treating the inpatients, both in rural and urban areas. A steady decline in use of Government sources and corresponding increase in private sources was evident (Fig. 15.2b).

Hospital Administration/Management

Hospital has an organization to organize and manage high quality patient care services (medical and nursing) which include acute

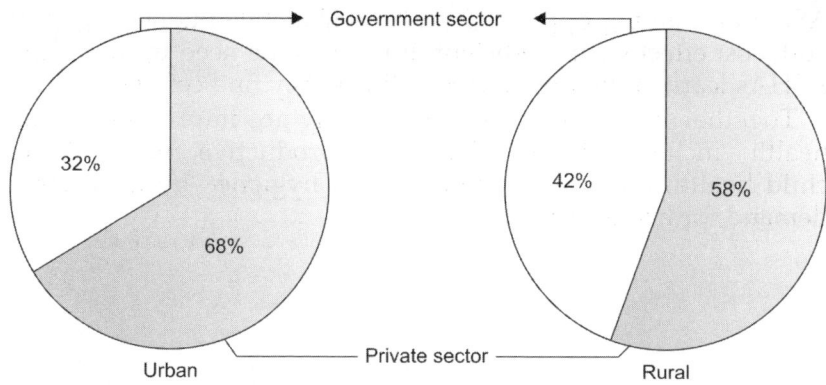

Fig. 15.2b: Indoor care services

patient care or emergency services, OPD, Indoor, laboratory services besides supportive services (Blood Bank, Laundary CSSD, Dietary, waste-management and infection control, maintaining patient records, cleanliness, and dispensing of drugs and materials, etc.). The hospital management comprise of planning of preventive, promotive, curative and rehabilitative services, managing human resources, materials and logistics and financial resources. Hospital designs and hospital engineering services are other important areas. Medical care in the hospitals is very costly inspite of Government Policy of free essential drugs, free diagnostics, free emergency and trauma services and free maternal and child care services and services for national health programmes. Hospital morbidity and mortality data is quality data for planning and evaluation of services.

KILKARI AND MOBILE ACADEMY—LAUNCHED IN 2016

KILKARI

Which means a baby's gurgle, delivers free weekly, time appropriate 72 audio messages about pregnancy, child health, child care directly to families mobile phones from the second trimester of pregnancy until the child is one year old. Kilkari has been launched in Jharkhand, Odisha, Uttar Pradesh, Uttarakhand and high priority districts of MP and Rajasthan state.

Mobile Academy

It is a free audio training course designed to expand and refresh the knowledge base of Accredited Social Health Activists (ASHAs) and improve their communication skills. Mobile Academy offers

ASHAs a training opportunity via their mobile phones which is both cost effective and efficient. It reduces the need to travel and ASHAs learn at their own pace at times they find convenient.

Together kilkari and mobile academy are improving family health—including family planning, reproductive, maternal and child health, nutrition, sanitation and hygiene—by generating demand for health services.

16

Occupational Safety and Health

Employee State Insurance Scheme (ESIS) coverage of employes: The wage ceiling has been raised from 15000 to 21000 ₹ per month with effect from 1st January 2017. Employees in receipt of daily average wage up to ₹ 100 per day are exempted from payment of contribution but entitled for benefits.

Under ESIS only employees who earn ₹ 21000 per month are covered, whereas the high wage earners are excluded from participation. It is a classic case of poor subsidizing for poorest and not necessarily the most equitable.

18

Infection Management and Environment Plan—Biomedical Waste Management

KAYAKALP—AN INITIATIVE FOR AWARDING PUBLIC HEALTH FACILITIES—LAUNCHED IN OCT 2014

Kayakalp initiative has been launched to promote cleanliness, hygiene and infection control practices in public health facilities as a part of Swachh Bharat Abhiyan. Under this initiative, public health care facilities shall be appraised and public health care facilities that show exemplary performance meeting standards protocols of cleanliness, hygiene and infection control will receive awards and commendation. It focuses on promoting cleanliness. Hygiene is critical to prevent nosocomial infections (Hospital acquired infections) as also a platform to **behavior change communication** in respect of environment. As a first principle of health care is "to do no harm" it is essential to have our health care facilities clean and ensure adherence to infection control practices. Best district hospital, best CHC and PHC are being awarded cash awards under NHM based on scoring system on the following parameters:

    i. Hospital facility upkeep

   ii. Sanitation and hygiene

  iii. Waste-management

  iv. Infection control

   v. Hygiene promotion

Ref: National Health Mission "Kayakalp" rejuvenating public health care facilities MOH and FW GOI 2015.

Index